Partnership and Pragmatism

Partnership and Pragmatism: Germany's response to AIDS prevention and care provides a comprehensive overview of the most important themes in German HIV/AIDS prevention and care from the beginning of the epidemic to the present. Multidisciplinary in approach, this book highlights the unique contributions of Germany to AIDS work, making available for the first time knowledge which can be applied to other countries as well as to other fields of public health practice. The innovative contributions included in this volume describe:

- *structural prevention*, a concept which unites political and behavioural change
- the synchronistic relationship between AIDS policy and gay politics
- the dominance of love and intimacy over other 'risk factors'
- an approach to prevention among drug users which emphasizes human rights and accepts the using behaviour
- a unique partnership between public authorities and the voluntary sector
- services for women working in cross-national border prostitution
- an AIDS survivor syndrome among gay men
- HIV in the context of emotional risks taken by women in relationships.

In addition, specifically German themes are described in detail, including the special needs of gay men from the former East Germany, the difficulties of providing adequate outpatient care for people with HIV/AIDS and the history of the AIDS prevention debate in Germany.

Offering medical, nursing, public health, sociological, psychological and social work perspectives on the German response to AIDS, this book provides a valuable source of reference for researchers, teachers and professionals working in AIDS prevention and care.

Rolf Rosenbrock is Professor of Public Health Policy at the Technical University of Berlin and Head of the Research Unit 'Public Health' at the Social Science Research Centre, Berlin. **Michael T. Wright** has been involved in HIV prevention since 1984 in the US and Germany and recently published *New International Directions in HIV Prevention for Gay and Bisexual Men* with B. R. Simon Rosser and Onno de Zwart.

Social aspects of AIDS
Series editor: Peter Aggleton
Institute of Education, University of London

AIDS is not simply a concern for scientists, doctors and medical researchers, it has important social dimensions as well. These include individual, cultural and media responses to the epidemic, stigmatisation and discrimination, counselling, care and health promotion. This series of books brings together work from many disciplines including psychology, sociology, cultural and media studies, anthropology, education and history. The titles will be of interest to the general reader, those involved in education and social research, and scientific researchers who want to examine the social aspects of AIDS.

Recent titles include:

Imagine Hope
Simon Watney

AIDS in Europe
New challenges for the social sciences
Edited by Jean-Paul Moatti, Yves Souteyrand, Annick Prieur, Theo Sandfort and Peter Aggleton

Dying to Care?
Work, stress and burnout in HIV/AIDS
David Miller

Mental Health and HIV Infection
Edited by José Catálan

The Dutch Response to HIV
Pragmatism and consensus
Edited by Theo Sandfort

Families and Communities Responding to AIDS
Edited by Peter Aggleton, Graham Hart and Peter Davies

Men Who Sell Sex
International perspectives on male prostitution and AIDS
Edited by Peter Aggleton

Sexual Behaviour and HIV/AIDS in Europe
Comparisons of national surveys
Edited by Michel Hubert, Nathalie Bajos and Theo Sandfort

Drug Injecting and HIV Infection
Global dimensions and local responses
Edited by Gerry Stimson, Don C. Des Jarlais and Andrew Ball

AIDS as a Gender Issue
Edited by Lorraine Sherr, Catherine Hankins and Lydia Bennett

AIDS
Activism and alliances
Edited by Peter Aggleton, Peter Davies and Graham Hart

Sexual Interactions and HIV Risk
New conceptual perspectives in European research
Edited by Luc van Campenhoudt, Mitchell Cohen, Gustavo Guizzardi and Dominique Hausser

Bisexualities and AIDS
International perspectives
Edited by Peter Aggleton

Crossing Borders
Migration, ethnicities and AIDS
Edited by Mary Haour-Knipe

Last Served?
Gendering the HIV pandemic
Cindy Patton

Moral Threats and Dangerous Desires
AIDS in the news media
Deborah Lupton

Power and Community
Organizational and cultural responses to AIDS
Dennis Altman

Partnership and Pragmatism

Germany's response to
AIDS prevention and care

**Edited by Rolf Rosenbrock and
Michael T. Wright**

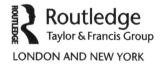

LONDON AND NEW YORK

First published 2000
by Routledge
711 Third Avenue, New York, NY 10017

Simultaneously published in the USA and Canada
by Routledge
2 Park Square, Milton Park, Abingdon, Oxfordshire OX14 4RN

Routledge is an imprint of the Taylor and Francis Group, an informa business

First issued in paperback 2015

© 2000 selection and editorial matter, Rolf Rosenbrock and Michael T.
Wright; individual chapters, the contributors.

Typeset in Times
by Curran Publishing Services Ltd, Norwich

British Library Cataloguing in Publication Data
A catalogue record for this book is available
from the British Library.

Library of Congress Cataloging in Publication Data
  Partnership and Pragmatism: Germany's response to AIDS prevention
  and care/[edited by] Rolf Rosenbrock and Michael T. Wright
  272 pp. 15.6 x 23.4 cm
  Includes bibliographical references and index
  1. AIDS (Disease) – Germany. I. Rosenbrock, Rolf. II. Wright, Michael T.
  RA644.A25 P3724 2000
  362.1'969792'00943—dc 21   00-031133

ISBN 978-0-415-24105-2 (hbk)
ISBN 978-1-138-88142-6 (pbk)

Contents

Figures

Tables

Contributors

Heinrich W. Ahlemeyer is the Executive Director of Sistema Consulting, a firm specialising in organisational development and management consulting. He is trained in organisational sociology (Bielefeld, Kiel, Münster, and Los Angeles) and management consulting (*Beratergruppe Neuwaldegg* in Vienna) and worked as a researcher from 1977–88. He is a lecturer in sociology at the University of Münster and Visiting Professor for Organisational Sociology at the University of Vienna. The focus of his work is organisational leadership, coaching for boards of directors, and corporate culture.

Gundula Barsch is Professor for Drug Use and Social Work Practice at a college in Merseburg (*Fachhochschule Merseburg*). She has carried out research in East Berlin on changes in illegal drug use during the period just after the Wall fell (1990–4). From 1994–8 she was director of the Department for Drug Users and People in Prison at the Deutsche AIDS-Hilfe, the national German AIDS organisation, working closely with the leadership of akzept (the National German Association for an Accepting Approach in Work with Drug Users and a Humane Drug Policy).

Michael Bochow is a research fellow at Intersofia, Berlin (Institute for Applied Interdisciplinary Research in Social Problems). Since 1987 he has been commissioned by the Federal Centre for Health Education (BZgA) and the Federal Ministry for Health to conduct nationwide studies of HIV risk behaviour among gay and bisexual men in Germany. His last book was about gay men in rural areas and smaller towns, taking Lower Saxony as an example (*Schwules Leben in der Provinz*, edition sigma, Berlin, 1998).

Martin Dannecker is Professor for the Study of Sexuality at the University of Frankfurt. His research and publications have focused on male homosexuality. Since 1987 he has examined prevention issues as well as the influence of AIDS on the sexual behaviour and lifestyles of homosexual men.

Willy H. Eirmbter is Professor for Sociology at the University of Trier. He has been involved since 1990 in research concerning lay concepts of AIDS and the impact of HIV/AIDS on social behaviour. He is now engaged in a research project sponsored by the DFG, investigating lay concepts of disease in general.

Stefan Etgeton is Executive Director of the Deutsche AIDS-Hilfe, the national German AIDS organisation, which is a federation of approximately 125 AIDS service organisations in Germany. After studying theology, philosophy and cultural science he wrote his dissertation in cultural science on 'The Text of Incarnation'. He has been politically active concerning a variety of issues.

Günter Frankenberg is a professor at the University of Frankfurt, currently holding the Chair for Administrative and Constitutional Law, the Philosophy of Law and Comparative Law. He has numerous publications, including work in the area of public health policy and the law.

Alois Hahn is Professor of Sociology at the University of Trier. He has carried out research on lay concepts of AIDS together with Willy H. Eirmbter and Rüdiger Jacob since 1990 and now is engaged in a research project sponsored by the DFG, investigating lay concepts of disease in general.

Alexander Hanebeck is a researcher assigned to the Chair for Administrative and Constitutional Law, the Philosophy of Law and Comparative Law at the University of Frankfurt.

Cornelia Helfferich is Professor for Sociology at the Protestant University of Applied Sciences in Freiburg and Director of the Institute for Social Science Research on Women (*Sozialwissenschaftliches Frauenforschungsinstitut – SoFFI*). She has carried out research on gender and health, with a focus on reproductive and sexual health and women's biographies.

Rainer Herrn is trained in both the natural and social sciences. He has conducted research on HIV prevention, the history of sexual science, and also on topics related to behavioural theory. He was a co-founder of the AIDS service movement in East Germany. Since 1991 he has headed the Research Post on the History of Sexual Science at the Humboldt University of Berlin. Since 1997 he has been curator of the English language exhibit '100 Years of the Gay Movement in Germany' sponsored by the Goethe Institute. From 1996–8 he was a researcher at the Social Science Research Centre Berlin (WZB) in the Research Unit Public Health Policy.

Rüdiger Jacob is senior lecturer in the Department of Sociology at the University of Trier. He has carried out research on lay concepts of AIDS together with Willy H. Eirmbter and Alois Hahn since 1990 and now works on health reporting systems for Germany as a whole and for the Trier region.

Michael F. Kraus has worked as a researcher at SPI-Research in Berlin since 1987. He has been in charge of projects concerning the heterosexual transmission of HIV and athletic activities for people with HIV. For the last several years the focus of his work has been providing scientific support to the Umbrella Network, a project funded by the European Commission.

Ulrich Marcus started his professional career at the Robert Koch Institute in Berlin in 1984. He began in the laboratory for retrovirus diagnosis, later moving to the documentation department of the newly founded AIDS Centre in Berlin. He was later appointed to be in charge of communication for AIDS research funding. Currently he is head of the communications department of the Robert Koch Institute and editor of a monthly public health journal.

Dorle Miesala-Edel is a sociologist serving as Director of Social Science Research within the Department for the Prevention of Contagious Diseases/AIDS at the Federal Ministry for Health. She is also the Director of the National AIDS Advisory Committee (*Nationaler AIDS Beirat*).

Martin Moers is Professor of Nursing at a college in Osnabrück (*Fachhochschule Osnabrück*). From 1990–4 he worked in collaboration with Doris Schaeffer at the Social Science Research Centre Berlin (WZB) in the Research Unit Public Health Policy led by Rolf Rosenbrock. During that time he participated in a number of projects concerning the care of people with HIV and AIDS.

Elisabeth Pott has served as the Director of the Federal Centre for Health Education (BZgA) in Cologne since 1986. The BZgA is a government authority specialised in the field of health promotion, prevention and health education. Her responsibilities include managing the successful national AIDS prevention campaign started by the BZgA in 1987. She also speaks nationally and internationally on various topics of public health and social medicine.

Rolf Rosenbrock, an economist and social scientist, is Head of the Research Unit Public Health Policy at the Social Science Research Centre Berlin (WZB), and is Professor of Public Health Policy at the Technical University of Berlin. He has served as a member of several parliamentary committees on AIDS and health care reform, as a member of the Scientific Committee of the Eighth and Ninth World AIDS Conferences, and as Co-Chair for Social and Behavioural Science at the Twelfth World AIDS Conference 1998 in Geneva. He is currently a member of several national advisory boards concerning various health care issues.

Doris Schaeffer is a sociologist and an education researcher. She currently holds a chair in the Department of Health Sciences at the University of Bielefeld. Her work focuses on public health nursing, nursing science, health care research, chronic diseases, AIDS, and professionalisation and collaboration in the health care system.

Rainer Schilling was a co-founder of the Deutsche AIDS-Hilfe (DAH), the national German AIDS organisation. He worked as a volunteer at the AIDS service organisation in Munich (*Münchener AIDS-Hilfe*) until the summer of 1987 when he went on staff at the DAH in the area of HIV prevention and gay men. Since 1990 he has been responsible for primary prevention for gay, bisexual men and sex workers in the DAH.

Martina Schöps-Potthoff is a sociologist at the Federal Ministry for Health responsible for areas related to AIDS prevention, social science AIDS research and substance abuse.

Elfriede Steffan is a project manager at SPI-Research in Berlin. She has carried out research on women's health, prostitution and drug addiction. The focus of her work in recent years has been the founding, implementing, and evaluating of pilot projects in Europe for the prevention of HIV and other STDs. She has various publications concerning drug use, gender, and prostitution.

Michael T. Wright has been involved in HIV prevention since 1984 in the US and Germany, having served as a psychotherapist, program manager, clinical supervisor, researcher, workshop leader and consultant. He is also trained in public health (Harvard University) and is currently a doctoral candidate in the Institute for Prevention and Psychosocial Research at the Free University of Berlin. His publications include *New and International Directions in HIV Prevention for Gay and Bisexual Men* with B. R. Simon Rosser and Onno de Zwart (Haworth Press, 1998).

Acknowledgement

The editors wish to acknowledge the financial support of the German Federal Ministry for Health which made the production of this book possible.

Part I
Introduction

1 Pragmatism and partnership

An overview of this volume

Rolf Rosenbrock and Michael T. Wright

It has been a daunting task to bring together in one volume a selection of articles depicting the cultural, social, political and scientific debates which have characterised the HIV epidemic in Germany. In such a limited space it was impossible to include contributions from all the women and men who have shaped the discourse over the years. We believe we have succeeded, however, in assembling a collection of writing which offers an international readership insight into many of the primary issues raised by AIDS in Germany. In selecting the themes and authors for this book we were guided by two questions: what have been the major topics in Germany's attempt to manage the epidemic, and what has been uniquely or characteristically German in the approaches taken? The former question led us to opt for a wide range of authors and subjects so as to present the many facets of HIV in this country. The latter question helped us to focus on aspects which to this point have not been accessible to the larger international audience, given that the discussion has taken place predominantly in German. The result is the only overview of HIV and AIDS in Germany available in English, offering an ideal starting point for those interested in the subject.

Although the authors represent a large diversity of professional backgrounds, philosophical perspectives, and political motivations, an important theme tying together the various contributions – and AIDS work in Germany more generally – is that of partnership and pragmatism. The partnership is evident not only in the formal collaborative structures which have been established between government and the voluntary sector, the national and local levels, the primarily affected groups and public authorities, social science and prevention practice – to name but a few. One also finds partnership in terms of a hard-won consensus regarding a new paradigm for disease prevention which was first pioneered on a large scale during the AIDS crisis. This approach, which Rolf Rosenbrock *et al.* (Chapter 20) call the 'new public health' rejects control and containment measures in favour of community-based models, state support for self-help structures, and the inclusion of social minorities in the design and implementation of interventions. The innovation brought to public health by AIDS is not unique to Germany; however, the forms which innovation has taken, both in terms of research and practice, reflect larger historical and social themes in German society which can be found in the articles presented here.

The aspect of pragmatism represents a compelling unifying principle which was an important factor in bringing the various players together to organise HIV prevention in Germany in its present form. Although the German discourse about HIV and AIDS – and about most aspects of life in general, and politics in particular – continues to be characterised by German philosophical idealism with an emphasis on principle, the search for a pragmatic approach to the epidemic provided a focus and a direction for prevention which made innovation possible.

Part I provides the introduction. Chapter 1 offers an overview of the volume's contents and unifying themes. Chapter 2 presents a brief description of key concepts within the German social welfare and health care systems which make up the context in which HIV and AIDS first appeared in Germany. This latter chapter is a sort of primer on important aspects of life in Germany related to the issue of HIV for those having minimal experience with the country.

Part II, 'History, policy, and epidemiology', describes the primary characteristics of the spread of HIV in Germany (Marcus, Chapter 3) as well as the political and social history of the country's response to the epidemic (Frankenberg and Hanebeck, Chapter 4). This is followed by descriptions of the structure and role of the three major players in HIV prevention on the national level: the Ministry for Health (Miesala-Edel and Schöps-Potthoff, Chapter 5), the Federal Centre for Health Education (Pott, Chapter 6), and the Deutsche AIDS-Hilfe, the National German AIDS Organisation. The description of the latter is divided into a chapter on the history and role of the AIDS service movement (Schilling, Chapter 8) and one describing the theoretical basis for prevention work with the primarily affected groups; namely, *structural prevention* (Etgeton, Chapter 7). Etgeton argues that the "structural" barriers in society need to be addressed – for example, discrimination, income disparity, and culture difference – if prevention is to have long-lasting effect. These chapters as a whole offer the reader insight into the development of the structures for prevention in German, the underlying principles of their work, and the ways in which they have been explicitly designed to address different aspects of the epidemic. Of course, the problems inherent in these structures are also discussed by the authors, particularly in light of the changing epidemic and growing financial constraints.

Part III entitled 'Risk perception and decision making in safer sex', presents in Chapter 9 data from national samples which show how perception of HIV risk in the general population is related to popular theories of disease aetiology (Jacob, Eirmbter and Hahn). The authors demonstrate the importance of these theories in defining risk, and how common explanations for the spread of disease are affected by such sociodemographic characteristics as age, education and social status. Chapter 10 by Heinrich W. Ahlemeyer presents HIV risk in terms of the intimate relationship, arguing from a systemic perspective that prevention targeting the individual is not enough in order to address risk-taking in a couple. This focus on the psychosexual dynamics of HIV risk has been an important basis for the development of prevention in Germany, standing in contrast to approaches which emphasize identifying risk factors and promoting behavioural change at the individual level. The main question driving prevention research and practice in this country has been: what is the political, social and relational context of risk-taking and healthy behaviour as opposed to what are the psychological risk factors for those engaging in unsafe sex, and how can we intervene with these individuals? In this vein, Martin Dannecker (Chapter 11) has ironically labelled love itself as being a risk factor. Dannecker makes clear, from the perspective of depth psychology, that risk and illusion are inherent aspects of the intimate sexual relationship. The challenge is not to eradicate these, but to develop interventions which acknowledge and respect their necessity while informing couples of the dangers involved.

In Part IV, 'Responding to specific target groups', the chapters present several aspects concerning the segments of the population particularly targeted by prevention and care measures. Four chapters discuss homosexual men, the largest group affected by HIV in Germany. Michael Bochow (Chapter 12) presents data from the National Gay Press Survey, which has been conducted at regular intervals since 1987. He discusses trends within the gay population over time, including the growing phenomenon of men of lower socioeconomic status being disproportionately affected by the disease. Rainer Herrn (Chapter 13) examines the unique situation of gay men from eastern Germany since the Wall fell, discussing how the characteristics of the prior East German society necessitate different approaches to prevention in that part of the country. Michael T. Wright (Chapter 18) and Rolf Rosenbrock (Chapter 19) look at the interplay between collective gay life and the epidemic. Wright presents evidence suggesting trauma reactions among gay men due to their community being disproportionately affected by the disease. He argues that these reactions resemble the 'survivor syndrome' found among other populations collectively faced with unusually high levels of disease and death. Rosenbrock considers the interaction between gay politics and AIDS politics, proposing that the epidemic has brought both positive and negative results to the gay liberation movement in Germany.

Also within the section concerning specific target groups is the contribution by Gundula Barsch (Chapter 14) in which the pioneering approach to drug use made possible by the HIV epidemic is presented. This approach emphasizes harm reduction and acceptance of drug using as the basis for intervention and policy. The ramifications of this approach are revolutionising drug prevention and treatment services in Germany. Cornelia Helfferich (Chapter 15) discusses risk perception among heterosexually active women, based on the results of national samples. Her analysis places HIV risk in the context of the other risks inherent in relationships, demonstrating that the perception and management of HIV risk is based on a host of social and relational factors. The unique situation of female prostitutes working on the border of Germany and Eastern European countries is discussed by Elfriede Steffan and Michael Kraus (Chapter 16). They present the work of the Umbrella Project which is designed to provide prevention services to that population. Finally, Doris Schaeffer (Chapter 17) discusses people with HIV/AIDS and the problems they encounter within the health care system. She argues that long overdue reforms within home care in Germany along with other deficits have led to mixed results as the system has attempted to cope with the changing needs of this patient group.

In Part V, 'The future of AIDS policy and practice', Rolf Rosenbrock, Doris Schaeffer and Martin Moers (Chapter 20) examine the process of 'normalisation' of AIDS in Germany; that is, the way in which HIV/AIDS has increasingly moved from the status of being an exceptional illness to a treatable condition. The authors depict the challenge now facing the German preventative and curative care system to adapt the innovations in AIDS prevention and care to other diseases. This challenge is made all the more difficult by the trend to re-medicalise the AIDS discourse and to neglect primary prevention, both in terms of resources and public attention.

It is our hope that this book not only provides documentation of HIV and AIDS in Germany for the years to come, but that it meaningfully contributes to the debate in industrialised countries about what we can learn from the AIDS epidemic so as to improve the effectiveness of public health and patient care more generally.

2 AIDS in a German context

A primer

Michael T. Wright

When HIV arrived in Germany in the early 1980s, there was already a dynamic landscape of tradition, law and organisational structure shaping and re-shaping society's response to social and health care problems. It is not the intent here to take on the impossible task of describing in one chapter the intricacies of this landscape. However, in these few pages an attempt is made to offer a schematic map which points out some of the important landmarks along the way, thereby making the following chapters more readable. This will be done by presenting a series of terms alphabetised by their English translations. Each term will be defined in its own right and as it relates to the other entries. The symbol ➤ indicates that the word immediately following has its own entry. In some instances, the term is discussed explicitly by the authors in this volume. Where this is the case, the corresponding chapters are noted at the end of the entry. The terms included here represent important underlying assumptions and traditions which have shaped the response to HIV in Germany.

This chapter is meant to function as a reference within the course of reading the book as well to be a quick glossary of important terms for HIV in Germany, in general. For a more detailed description of the German health care system, the reader is referred to Knox (1993), Stone (1980), Rosenberg (1986), Webber (1992), Wysong and Abel (1996), and Kirkman-Liff (1990). An insightful comparison of the concept of solidarity (see definition below) as found in the US and Germany is offered by Reinhardt (1996).

AIDS Service Organisations (AIDS-Hilfen) The AIDS Service Organisations (ASOs) in Germany are voluntary organisations (non-profit making) with the mandate of providing various prevention and care services to the primarily affected groups. All ASOs receive the majority of their funding from public authorities and employ both paid and non-paid staff. Almost all ASOs are members of the ➤ Deutsche AIDS-Hilfe. (See Schilling, Chapter 8; Etgeton, Chapter 7; Frankenberg and Hanebeck, Chapter 4.)

Associations (Vereine, Verbände) There is no adequate English translation for the German words *Vereine* and *Verbände*, as these words denote particular organisational forms based in a specific cultural tradition. There is a joke which says that wherever three Germans are, there is at least one association. This alludes to the important role which clubs and associations of various sizes have within German society and to the cultural tendency to create formal organisations for each specific interest. Of course, associations of various sorts exist in all cultures where people are free to associate. Characteristically German, however, is the establishment of local, regional, and national chapters for each particular activity, with co-ordination structures and areas of responsibility being outlined for each organisational level. Already in 1983 the -> Deutsche AIDS-Hilfe was founded as the national organisation. Since that time over 120 other ⇾ AIDS Service Organisations (ASOs) have been founded and nearly all of them are members of the national organisation. Although each ASO is incorporated separately and is technically not obliged to follow recommendations from the national office, the cultural tendency to create unifying regional and national structures and to identify common principles has resulted in a co-ordinated, relatively uniform, and geographically comprehensive network of HIV prevention in the country.

Deutsche AIDS-Hilfe, the National German AIDS Organisation   The Deutsche AIDS-Hilfe (DAH), which translates literally as 'German AIDS Assistance', is the national federation of ⇾ AIDS service organisations (ASOs) in Germany. The DAH is a voluntary organisation funded almost entirely by the ⇾ Federal Ministry for Health through the ⇾Federal Centre for Health Education. The DAH has over 120 member ASOs which are themselves organised at the local and regional levels. The DAH acts as a lobby group for HIV at the national level, produces prevention concepts and materials for the primarily affected groups, and provides technical support for the work of its members. (See Schilling, Chapter 8; Etgeton, Chapter 7.)

Federal Centre for Health Education (Bundeszentrale für gesundheitliche Aufklärung, BZgA)   The Federal Centre for Health Education (BZgA) is a governmental organisation which was set up to be the official provider of prevention campaigns to the general public regarding a variety of health issues. The BZgA is funded by the ⇾ Federal Ministry for Health to conduct HIV prevention. The BZgA designs and implements campaigns at the national level for the general population and contracts with the ⇾ Deutsche AIDS-Hilfe to provide prevention and education for the primarily affected groups. (See Pott, Chapter 6.)

Federal Ministry for Health (Bundesministerium für Gesundheit, BMG)   The Federal Ministry for Health (BMG) is responsible for funding certain forms of prevention at the national level. This mandate is fulfilled by exclusive contracts with the ⇾ Federal Centre for Health Education (BZgA). In the case of HIV, the BZgA in turn provides funding to the ⇾ Deutsche AIDS-Hilfe. (See Miesala-Edel and Schöps-Potthoff, Chapter 5.)

Federalism (Föderalismus)   The post-war German constitution explicitly promotes a delegation of responsibilities for several areas of government, including social welfare and health care, to the sixteen federal states (or *Länder* as they are called in German) and to the local communities. This has meant, for example, that ⇢ AIDS service organisations are funded by their corresponding local or regional governmental body. Only the ⇢ Deutsche AIDS-Hilfe receives federal funding, given its national mandate. This commitment to decentralised government is, however, deceiving to the outsider, given the cultural tendency toward uniformity through the creation of regional and national ⇢ associations. In effect, the federalist structure plays the most important role in setting funding priorities; the actual service structures, however, are nationally co-ordinated and bear strong similarities across regions.

Gay movement (Schwulenbewegung)   The gay liberation movement in Germany began in the late nineteenth century, led by Magnus Hirschfeld and his contemporaries in Berlin. The budding gay and lesbian subcultures following the First World War were brutally repressed during the Nazi period. The movement reorganised in the post-war years, gaining particular strength in the late 1960s and during the 1970s. An important reason for the ⇢ AIDS service organisations being able to establish a response so early in the epidemic was the existing networks of formal and informal gay groups which had been established in the decades prior to the first AIDS cases. (See Rosenbrock, Chapter 19; Shilling, Chapter 8.)

Health insurance (Krankenversicherung)   Germany does not have a nationalised health care system with a central payer, but nevertheless achieves virtual universal coverage through a system of statutory health insurance funds which are part of a larger health care co-ordinating structure. These bodies – owned by the insured, self-administered by elected representatives, and acting under public law – are part of the ⇢ social insurance system, covering the vast majority of expenses in the health sector. HIV and related conditions have been covered by statutory health insurance funds, essentially ensuring access to care for people with HIV/AIDS. There are also private insurance companies which selectively admit members and pay according to stricter criteria; however, participation in these insurance programmes is voluntary and only open to people in higher income brackets and civil servants. (See Miesala-Edel and Schöps-Potthoff, Chapter 5.)

Host organisation (Träger)   Many social welfare and health care organisations have a host organisation which is the conduit for funding and ⇢ provider of the necessary infrastructure. The largest host organisations are the ⇢ Social Welfare Associations; however, many organisations do exist independently of a host organisation and receive funds directly (as in the case of many ⇢ AIDS service organisations). (See Schaeffer, Chapter 17; Miesala-Edel and Schöps-Potthoff, Chapter 5.)

Immigrant/foreigner (Migrant/Ausländer)   The segment of the German population with the sharpest increase in new AIDS cases in recent years is immigrants. The requirements for citizenship in Germany are unusually restrictive, as compared with other industrialised nations, favouring German ancestry over residency in the country. As a result, the term immigrant refers not only to those who have recently arrived in Germany, but also to many residents who were born to non-nationals and raised in the country. (See Marcus, Chapter 3.)

Social insurance system (Sozialversicherung)   A central feature of German social welfare and health care services is the social insurance system, analogous to programs in other industrialised countries. This system, formalised in the nine-teenth century and extensively expanded in the post-war period, includes work-related accident insurance, old age pension, unemployment insurance, ⇒ health insurance, and most recently, long-term care insurance for the severely ill. An important issue for people with HIV/AIDS has been the young age of infirmity. This has meant forced retirement on a very low pension or without a pension, given that those affected were two young to have paid substantially into the system. The addition of the long-term care insurance has meant the creation of new services for outpatient care, including services for people with HIV/AIDS; however, the resultant service structures have not been sufficient to meet the need. (See Schaeffer, Chapter 17.)

Social welfare associations (Verbände der Freien Wohlfahrtspflege)   Many social welfare and health care services in Germany are provided by the six Social Welfare Associations. Most of the organisations in the voluntary sector are somehow connected with one of these Associations, either by becoming Association members themselves, or through the membership of their ⇒ host organisations. The Social Welfare Associations represent the interests of the voluntary sector at the regional and national levels. By tradition, each of the Associations has specific areas of expertise; however, in actuality, there is consid-erable overlap in the types of services offered. The Social Welfare Associations act as conduits for funds, lobbying groups, and co-ordinating bodies. Local affiliates of the Associations can also act as ⇒ host organisations for the voluntary sector. These structures reflect the tradition of ⇒ associations more generally in Germany. (See Schaeffer, Chapter 17.)

Social welfare state (Sozialstaat)   The German word *Sozialstaat* can only approximately be rendered by the English phrase 'social welfare state'. Whereas, the latter is seen in many English-speaking countries as being aligned with a particular political ideology; the *Sozialstaat* is anchored in the post-war German constitution as being a fundamental characteristic of German government, standing alongside democracy, republican structures and the rule of law. The political question focuses not on whether Germany should be a social welfare state, but rather, how this mandate should be fulfilled. This strong social welfare tradition, protected in the constitution and codified in various legal forms, has provided an important foundation for the response to the HIV epidemic.

Essentially, the -> AIDS service organisations and other care structures were established on the basis of an already widely-accepted and institutionalised system of providing for those in need. Two important principles of the social welfare state are -> solidarity and -> subsidiarity.

Solidarity principle (Solidaritätsprinzip)   This guiding principle of the German -> social welfare state goes beyond the usual connotation of the word solidarity in English. The solidarity principle is more than empathy for others and symbolic or material acts of support at the individual level. It implies the duty of society as a whole, through its governmental and economic structures, to provide the necessary collective support in order to minimise the risks of financial, social, and physical harm and to compensate for the economic and social disadvantage experienced by certain segments of the population. This principle is not specific to left wing political parties, having its origins in social philosophy and Lutheran and Catholic social teaching. The principle of solidarity has been invoked in relation to HIV several times in order to muster support for discriminated minorities in their fight against the epidemic.

Structural prevention (strukturelle Prävention)   This is the primary concept underlying HIV prevention in Germany, particularly in working with the primarily affected groups. The concept was first coined and defined by the -> Deutsche AIDS-Hilfe. Based on the WHO Ottawa Charter, structural prevention rests on the premise that the "structural" barriers to health behaviour in society need to be addressed – for example, discrimination, income disparity, and cultural difference – if prevention is to have long lasting effect. In concrete terms, behaviour change at the individual level is made possible through changes in the social, political, and cultural contexts which affect health and risk behaviour. This implies that prevention work by definition has an explicit political component. (See Etgeton, Chapter 7.)

Subsidiarity principle (Subsidiaritätsprinzip)   This guiding principle of the German -> social welfare state has its origins in Catholic social teaching. The idea is that social problems should be dealt with at the lowest level of organisational complexity possible within the structures of society. For example, self-help is preferable to help from others and services organised and administered at the local level through voluntary organisations is preferable to interventions from the national government. The subsidiarity principle is not to be confused with the concepts of self-sufficiency and community work. These latter concepts, as found particularly in English-speaking countries, are based in traditions of individualism and decentralised government. Although the subsidiarity principle favours local initiative, the focus is not on the individual but rather on society. As the English word subsidiary also suggests, the parts are dependent on the whole. Therefore, it is in accordance with the principle of subsidiarity that public authorities fund self-help initiatives to act in their own interest, even if the political positions or the methods of the self-help groups do not exactly fit the ideology of the standing government. A good example are the ⇒ AIDS service organisations in Germany which have used public funding to produce sexually explicit prevention materials. The Government itself may not approve of the content *per se*, but if the materials prove to be effective for the target groups, then the principle of subsidiarity has been fulfilled and the direct intervention of the Government is unnecessary.

References

Kirkman-Liff, B. L. (1990) 'Physician payment and cost containment in West-Germany,' *Journal for Health Policy, Politics, and Law* 15(1): 69–99.

Knox, R. (1993) *Germany's Health System: One Nation, United with Health Care for All*, Washington, D.C.: Faulkner and Gray.

Reinhardt, U. E. (1996) 'A social contract for 21st century health care: three-tier health care with bounty hunting,' *Health Economics* 5: 479–99.

Rosenberg, P. (1986) 'The origin and the development of compulsory health insurance in Germany', in D. Light (ed.), *Political Values and Health Care: The German Experience*, Cambridge, Mass.: MIT Press.

Stone, D. A. (1980) *The Limits of Professional Power: National Health Care in the Federal Republic of Germany*, Chicago: University of Chicago Press.

Webber, D. (1992) 'The politics of regulatory change in the German health sector,' in K. Dyson (ed.), *The Politics of German Regulation*, Aldershot, UK: Dartmouth.

Wysong, J. A. and Abel, T. (1996) 'Risk equalation, competition, and choice: a preliminary assessment of the 1993 German health reform.", *Sozial- und Präventivmedizin* 41: 212–23.

Part II
History, policy and epidemiology

Part II

3   The epidemiology of HIV and AIDS in Germany

Ulrich Marcus

Introduction

Like in most other Western European countries the HIV epidemic in Germany began in the early 1980s. Though there may have been sporadic introductions of the virus into Germany from other sources, the epidemic began with the introduction of HIV into the gay communities of West Germany through men who had been infected through gay contacts on the East and West Coasts of the US.

During the 1970s openly gay communities had developed in the large West German cities, especially in West Berlin, Hamburg, Munich, Frankfurt and Cologne. These communities – with their infrastructure of cafés, bars, discotheques, bath houses and non-commercial meeting points – facilitated the search for partners and for sex. But the lifestyle which developed in the gay subcultures of the larger cities unfortunately also facilitated the spread of sexually transmitted diseases such as gonorrhoea, syphilis and hepatitis B.

Compared with the US the epidemic spread of HIV in Western Europe was delayed by about two to four years. The course of the epidemic among gay men in the various European countries was shaped by the time the virus was introduced and by the degree of geographical concentration of the gay communities. Gay life was highly concentrated in the largest cities of France (Paris), the UK (London), Denmark (Copenhagen), Sweden (Stockholm), The Netherlands (Amsterdam) and Switzerland (Zurich). In Germany – and to a similar extent also in Italy and Spain – the gay communities were more dispersed into several, equally important centres. This may have slowed the initial spread of HIV in these demographically less centralised countries.

Concerning drug policy, Germany followed a strategy which was less permissive than the very liberal Dutch approach, but also less restrictive than that of the French and the Americans, the US having the most repressive 'War on Drugs' policy. A network of drug counselling and social service centres had already been established in the larger cities, engaging in secondary prevention activities among drug users. The general social and political climate favoured the idea of drug abuse as a social and health problem as opposed to being a criminal offence.

The medical and public health systems were hardly prepared to deal with an emerging HIV epidemic. The epidemiology and prevention of infectious diseases

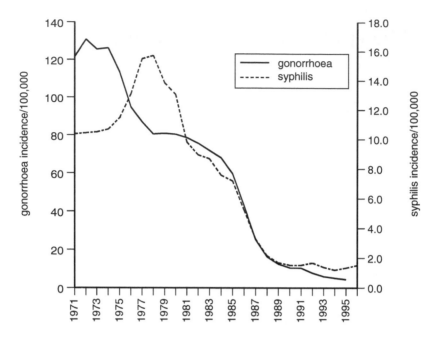

Figure 3.1 Gonorrhoea and syphilis in western Germany, 1971–96

Note: The different levels of incidence in Figures 3.1, 3.2 and 3.3 may not reflect real differences, because the extent of under-reporting may differ. Note also different scales.

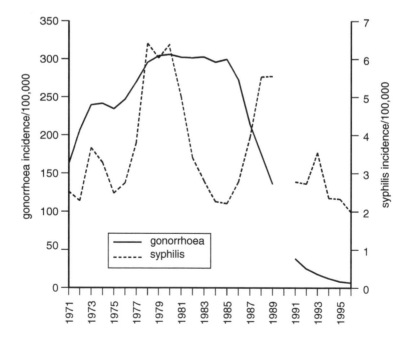

Figure 3.2 Gonorrhoea and syphilis incidence in eastern Germany, 1971–96

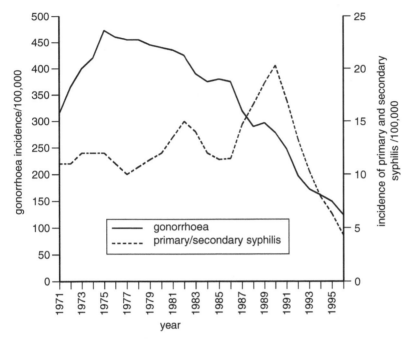

Figure 3.3 Gonorrhoea and syphilis in the US, 1971–96

had been neglected because of the prevailing notion that these diseases were either easily prevented by vaccines or easily treated by antibiotics, thus not requiring special attention.

The first responses to the emerging epidemic

Because the traditional actors, such as the public health system and the curative medical system, were unable or unwilling to develop a concept for the primary prevention of a sexually transmitted, fatal virus infection primarily affecting marginalised communities, a brave political decision was taken. For the first time in the public health policy of post-war Germany, grass-root organisations – in this case gay men – were allowed to play a central role in the prevention activities that were set up to deal with the emerging problem. (See Frankenberg and Hanebeck, Chapter 4, for a description of the policy debate; Schilling, Chapter 8 and Rosenbrock, Chapter 19, for the role of the AIDS service organisations and the gay community.)

The risk-group oriented prevention efforts were complemented by an 'umbrella' campaign for the general population. This campaign was executed by federal and state agencies and focused not only on promoting condoms, but also on disseminating information on HIV transmission and promoting solidarity with those affected by the disease. (See Pott, Chapter 6, regarding the campaigns for the general population and Miesela-Edel and Schöps-Potthoff, Chapter 5, regarding the division of prevention activities between the governmental and voluntary sectors.)

The epidemic becomes visible

Thanks to contact with the research team of Robert Gallo in the US, the Robert Koch Institute in Berlin was already conducting HIV surveillance studies with antibody test kits in autumn 1984, among the first institutions world-wide to do so (see Pauli *et al.*, 1985). The results were alarming: HIV antibodies were detected in approximately 60 per cent of haemophiliacs, 35 per cent of gay men, and 22 per cent of intravenous drug users tested. Though it was questionable how representative these numbers were, it was obvious that the virus was spreading quickly. In the absence of systematically collected data, early estimates of the size of the epidemic (later found to be exaggerated) based on these first surveillance studies estimated the number of persons already infected in West Germany at around 100,000.

The epidemiological surveillance system

In the following years a surveillance system was established which consists of a voluntary anonymous reporting scheme for AIDS cases, a mandatory anonymous reporting scheme for laboratories performing HIV confirmation testing, a sentinel surveillance system for HIV and other STDs (starting in 1988), analysis of the screening results from blood donors, anonymous unlinked testing of new-borns in two states (Berlin and Lower Saxony), an additional sentinel study in the new eastern German states (the former East Germany), prevalence studies among certain groups, and research on the incidence of HIV and the occurrence of risk behaviour among gay men and IV drug users.

The AIDS case registry can be validated quantitatively to some extent by counterchecking with the cause of death register. (In Germany checking individual reports is not legally possible for data security and confidentiality reasons.) The quantitative comparison of these two data sources shows that about 85 per cent of all AIDS cases are actually reported within the existing voluntary anonymous system.

The surveillance system paints the following picture of the HIV epidemic in Germany. As of the end of 1998 a cumulated total of 17,995 AIDS cases had been reported in the AIDS register. A total of 88.4 per cent of these cases were diagnosed in men and 11.6 per cent in women. About 75 per cent of the reported cases are already deceased. Comprising almost two-thirds of all cases, gay men are the largest group among people with AIDS. They are followed by IV drug users (15 per cent) and those infected through heterosexual intercourse (6 per cent). Foreign residents from high-prevalence countries are in a separate category, most of them having been infected by unprotected heterosexual intercourse. Since epidemiological patterns in this group are generally reflective of the distribution of HIV in their countries of origin, it makes sense to count this group separately.

The median age of all AIDS patients at the time of diagnosis is 39 years. The median age is highest among transfusion recipients (49.4 years), followed by gay/bisexual men (40.1 years), heterosexuals (*c.* 40 years), IV drug users (33.4 years), and foreign residents from high-prevalence countries (31.6 years).

Up to the end of 1998 laboratories reported more than 130,000 confirmed antibody positive test results. Due to the anonymous reporting system and the lack of unique identifiers, this number contains a considerable amount of double counting. Only since 1993 are labs asked to identify which of the tests are known to be primary diagnoses. The number of explicitly identified new HIV diagnoses during the last five years has been around 2,000–2,500 per year, only about one-third of all lab reports.

Taking into account the relatively constant level of newly-diagnosed HIV infections during the 1990s and calculating the course and extent of the epidemic during the 1980s by back calculation models based on the number and course of AIDS diagnoses, the number of people currently living in Germany with HIV and AIDS can be estimated at about 42,000. Approximately 20,000 persons already have died from AIDS since the beginning of the epidemic in Germany. These estimates fit well with the sentinel data which estimate the number of people with HIV and AIDS receiving medical care in 1994 at 24,000.

The German HIV/AIDS epidemic in the European context

Comparing Germany with Northern European countries (for example, Belgium, The Netherlands, Denmark and the UK) the course and extent of the epidemic is very similar. A comparable course, but with higher prevalence levels, can be observed in France and Switzerland. In Italy, Spain and Portugal the epidemic

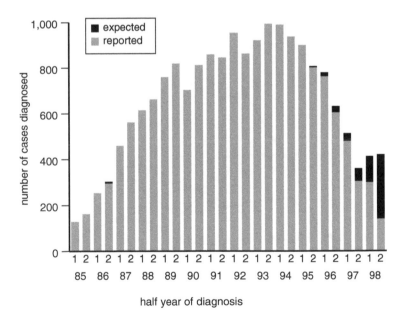

Figure 3.4 AIDS cases in Germany by half year of diagnosis, adjusted for reported delays

Note: The decline since 1995 is mainly due to the inproved therapeutic options and the earlier start of therapy.

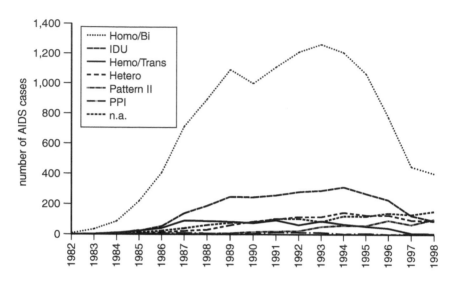

Figure 3.5 AIDS cases by means of transmission and year of diagnosis

Note: In all subsequent figures:

    PPI = pre/perinatal infection

    Pattern II = persons from high prevalence regions (sub-Saharan Africa, parts of Southeast
                    Asia and the Carribean)

    n.a. = information not available

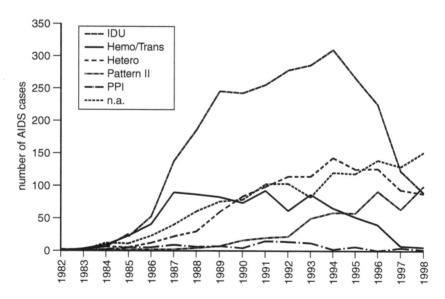

Figure 3.6 Number of cases by means of transmission and year of diagnosis,
             homosexuals excluded

Note: The only groups in which AIDS diagnoses have not declined since 1995 are among people
      from Pattern II regions and those for whom no information on transmission risk is available.

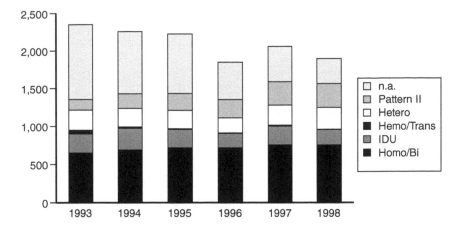

Figure 3.7 HIV infections by means of transmission and year of diagnosis

began a bit later, with the number of AIDS cases initially increasing more steeply then levelling off in more recent years (European Centre, quarterly reports).

The differences between Germany and countries with higher AIDS incidence rates are mainly attributable to a differing dynamic of the epidemic among IV drug users and heterosexuals, as will be discussed below.

The HIV epidemic among gay men

The epidemic among gay men is mainly concentrated in the five largest metropolitan areas: Berlin, Frankfurt, Hamburg, Munich and Cologne/Düsseldorf. More than 60 per cent of all AIDS cases among gay men have been diagnosed in these five areas. The majority of new infections in this group continues to occur in these cities.

Looking at the age distribution among newly-diagnosed HIV-positive gay men, no obvious downward trend to younger age groups can be identified. But there is a clear socially downward trend; that is, the proportion of gay men from lower socio-economic strata of the population is increasing among newly-infected persons.

The HIV epidemic among IV drug users

The most striking difference in the epidemiological development between northern European countries (including Germany) and southern European countries (including France and Switzerland) is the extent of the epidemic among IV drug users. The fact that the IV drug user epidemic has been contained in Germany is the main reason for the comparatively small number of heterosexually-infected persons, since in developed countries sexual contact

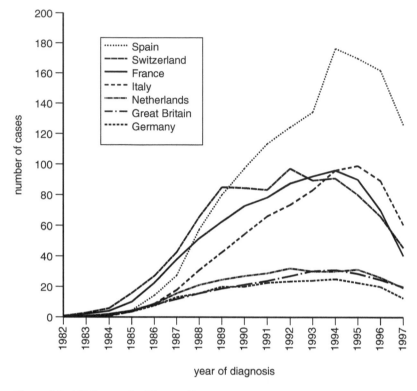

Figure 3.8 AIDS cases / million residents

with IV drug users has long been the main source of heterosexually-acquired HIV infections. One very important reason for the successful containment of the HIV epidemic among drug users was the early implementation of harm reduction measures like needle exchange schemes and relatively easy access to drug injection equipment. It is, however, interesting how similar the rates of reported needle-sharing among drug users can be in countries with widely differing dynamics within their respective IV drug user epidemics. Possible explanations for this may be the point in time when prevention efforts were initiated, the extent of adjustments in risk-taking behaviours among drug users due to knowledge of their HIV status, and socio-cultural differences among drug users in different countries which may affect the settings of drug-taking and the associated transmission risks.

The HIV epidemic among recipients of blood and blood products

Before 1985 blood donations were not screened for HIV; and blood components, like clotting factor concentrates for the treatment of haemophiliacs, were only partially heat-inactivated. Therefore, blood transfusions and

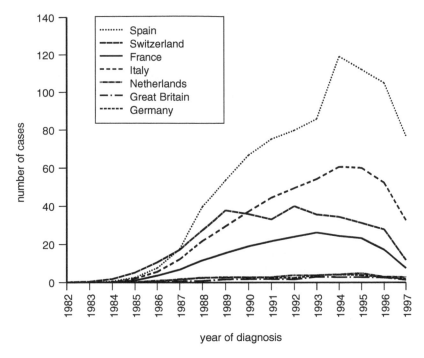

year of diagnosis

Figure 3.9 AIDS cases among IDU / million residents

treatment with blood components could result in transmission of HIV. Because the clotting factor concentrates used for treatment of German haemophiliacs were largely imported from the US, where HIV was already spreading in the donor population since the early 1980s, a large number of haemophiliacs became infected with HIV even before the problem was recognised and could be addressed. Retrospective testing of blood samples from haemophiliacs as well as back-calculation models show that the large majority of HIV infections among haemophiliacs was already acquired by 1983–4. In Germany discussions about the possible risk of transmission of HIV through blood and blood components started in 1983. The first action that was taken was the exclusion of so called 'risk group' donors from the donor population; namely, homosexual men and intravenous drug users. Donor screening for HIV and heat inactivation for clotting factor concentrates were introduced in 1985. Up to that point about 1,300 haemophiliacs in Germany had been infected with HIV; almost 600 died by the end of 1998. Only a handful of haemophiliacs from East Germany became infected with HIV, since clotting factors were produced from their own donor population (as in all Eastern European countries and in some Western European countries; for example, Belgium, the Netherlands and Finland).

The course and extent of the HIV epidemic among haemophiliacs from the countries which used commercially available clotting factor concentrates produced in the US show little variation, with the exception of Spain, where those products were used longer and more intensely than in the other European countries. Also the HIV epidemic among transfusion recipients, which more closely reflects the spread of HIV in the respective national blood donor populations, is very similar across Europe. An exception is France. Because of the French HIV blood contamination scandal, several high ranked officials and politicians (including the prime minister at the time) were charged with negligence. They were accused of postponing donor screening with US antibody tests while waiting for the production of French-made test kits, which only became available some months later. In point of fact, donor screening was introduced in France and other European countries almost at the same time (in the middle of 1985). The main reason for the more serious transfusion-related HIV epidemic in France is probably due not to a delayed introduction of donor screening, but rather to a higher prevalence of HIV in the donor population (Hamers, 1996). It is worth mentioning in this regard that donor selection, as it was introduced in Germany and other European countries in 1983, was not practised in France until 1987. Until then it was usual practice to collect blood donations in prisons, for example, regardless of the considerably high percentage of drug users in that population.

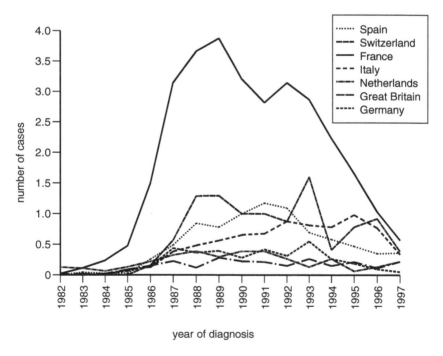

Figure 3.10 AIDS cases among transfusion recipients / million residents

The heterosexual HIV epidemic

The spread of HIV by heterosexual contacts has remained quite limited thus far. Until 1997 only 6 per cent of all AIDS patients had been infected by heterosexual intercourse, though the percentage increased from 2.3 per cent before 1988 to 9 per cent in 1998. Heterosexual transmission is much more prevalent in females than in males. Sources of infection for females are generally drug-using partners, bisexual partners, partners from high-prevalence countries, partners with haemophilia, and transfusion recipients.

So far, very few men have been infected by intercourse with women. Their female partners have generally been women from high prevalence countries, drug-using women, women who have been infected via heterosexual intercourse, and transfusion recipients.

A considerable and growing percentage of heterosexual AIDS patients is unable to provide information on the transmission risk of their HIV-infected partners. Regardless of this phenomenon, surveillance data so far do not support the existence of an independent, emerging HIV epidemic among the heterosexual population in Germany. This can be attributed to the successful containment of the HIV epidemic among drug users. It is not coincidental that the highest AIDS incidence among heterosexuals is found in those European countries which also have the highest AIDS incidence rates among intravenous drug users. Since an autonomous heterosexual HIV epidemic has not developed so far in Germany, the importation of HIV infections via unprotected intercourse with persons from high prevalence parts of the world plays a significant role for the heterosexual

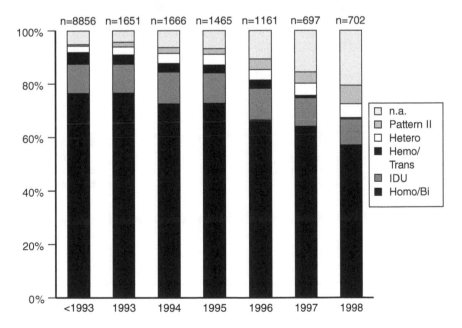

Figure 3.11 Means of transmission for male AIDS cases

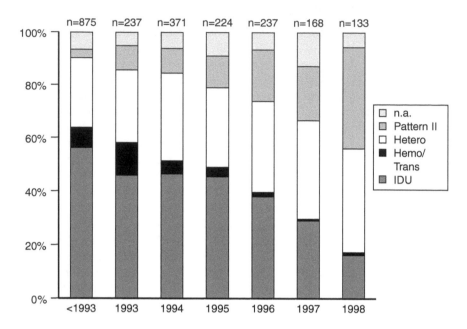

Figure 3.12 Means of transmission for female AIDS cases

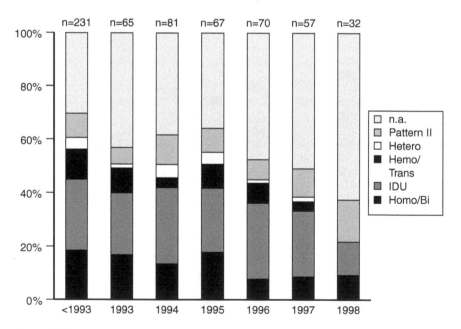

Figure 3.13 Means of transmission for the male partner of heterosexually-infected female AIDS cases

transmission of HIV: whether abroad through 'sex tourism' or by contact to nationals from these regions residing in Germany.

AIDS and HIV infection in women

The German HIV epidemic is still very much male-dominated, since three of the largest affected groups (homosexual men, intravenous drug users and immigrants from high prevalence countries) consist exclusively or largely of men. Female prostitutes, who in high prevalence parts of the world are one of the groups with the greatest risk of infection, are so far hardly affected by HIV in Germany. (The exception is prostitutes using intravenous drugs whose source of infection is generally needle-sharing rather than unprotected intercourse with clients.) One of the reasons for this is a high degree of professionalism among the women who work as prostitutes, which enables them to achieve a high rate of condom use in commercial sexual encounters (Velten and Kleiber, 1994; Markert, 1994). Another reason might be a lower frequency of prostitution contacts in a developed country, such as Germany, as compared to developing countries. This could be related to socio-cultural and socio-economic differences, like higher numbers of migrant workers in the developing world. Also the rate of other sexually transmitted diseases which may favour the acquisition of HIV is generally lower in developed countries (Gerbase *et al.*, 1998).

Nevertheless, the transmission risks for women have changed during the course of the epidemic. While during the first years the majority of HIV infections in women were due to drug use related risks, currently most infections are transmitted through heterosexual intercourse. Also, the number of women who are unaware of the risks taken by their partners is steadily increasing. Among newly-diagnosed HIV infections the percentage of women has risen to 20 per cent, a level reached at the beginning of the 1990s which has since remained unchanged. The median age of HIV infection for women is considerably lower than for men (median age at time of AIDS diagnosis for men 38 years, for women 32 years).

With a growing number of HIV-infected women of child-bearing age one might expect an increase of perinatally-infected children. Contrary to these expectations the number of perinatal HIV cases is decreasing. In general, mother-to-child transmission of HIV plays a minor role in developed countries as compared to developing countries, because the reproduction rate is lower (Stephenson *et al.*, 1996; De Vincenzi *et al.*, 1997). Exaggerated expectations concerning the rate of transmission to the child and the lack of medical interventions to prevent transmission resulted in high rates of pregnancy termination in the first years of the epidemic (Lutz-Friedrich, 1999). Since 1994 the situation has changed. In that year the ACTG 076 trial showed that zidovudine therapy during pregnancy reduced the risk of transmission to the child considerably (Connor *et al.*, 1994). At the same time, the retrospective analysis of the German data on the mode of delivery revealed that caesarean section before the start of labour reduced the risk of transmission, as well (Schaefer *et al.*, 1994).

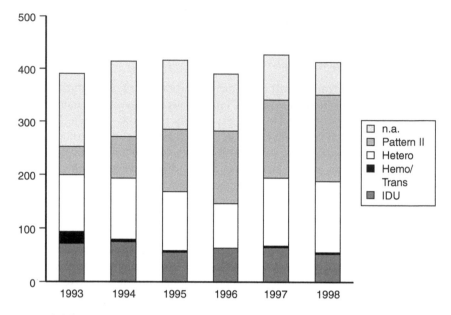

Figure 3.14 HIV infections in women by means of transmission and year of diagnosis

Thus several years before caesarean section was internationally accepted as a means to reduce the mother-to-child transmission rate, the combination of anti-retroviral treatment with zidovudine and delivery by caesarean section was established as the standard practice in Germany to prevent transmission, leading to a mother-to-child transmission rate of below 2 per cent. Currently the number of HIV-infected new-borns is estimated to be below ten cases per year. Most transmissions are due to the failure to detect HIV infection in the mother before or during pregnancy.

The development of the HIV/AIDS epidemic in the former East Germany

Before the reunification of the country in 1990, HIV had not spread very far in the former East Germany. By 1989 only nineteen cases of AIDS had been diag-nosed in East Germany and a total of less than 100 HIV infections had been detected in the entire country. The limited spread of HIV can be explained by the restrictions for citizens wanting to travel outside the country, a lesser degree of mobility within the country itself, the lack of an intravenous drug using popu-lation, and a different lifestyle within the gay community characterised by a poorly developed infrastructure of bars and other exclusively gay meeting places, the absence of gay bath houses and backroom bars, and relatively closed social and sexual networks. Most of these conditions changed with the reunification. (See Herrn, Chapter 13.)

Contrary to the situation in West Germany in the beginning of the 1980s, it was known by the time the Wall fell how HIV was transmitted and how transmission could be avoided. Thus, although the pace of the epidemic in eastern Germany accelerated after reunification, HIV did not spread as rapidly as in West Germany in the early 1980s. Since intravenous drug use is still largely absent from eastern Germany, homosexual men are by far the largest affected group. Especially in Berlin, where the heavily-affected gay community from the western part of the city mixed with the minimally-affected gay community from the East, the large gap between the prevalence rates is closing, but has not yet disappeared completely.

AIDS and HIV among foreign residents living in Germany

Within the European Union, Germany has been one of the countries with the most restrictive naturalisation laws. Therefore, the foreign nationals living in Germany are not only those who immigrated recently, but also a large number of children who were born and grew up in Germany, but whose parents immigrated from another country.

The percentage of AIDS patients without German citizenship is 15 per cent, while the share of non-German citizens in the whole population is 8.9 per cent. AIDS has been diagnosed in persons from 123 countries, more than half of them (55 per cent) being from other European countries, Turkey included. Patients from outside of Europe come from Sub-Saharan Africa (39 per cent), the Americas (North 26 per cent, South 13 per cent) and Asia (18 per cent).

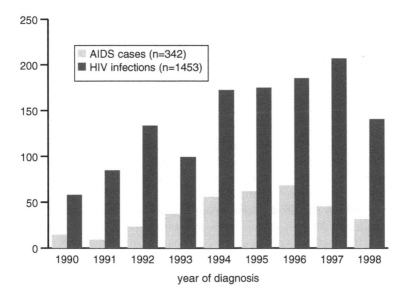

Figure 3.15 Number of AIDS and HIV diagnoses in eastern Germany after the reunification in 1990

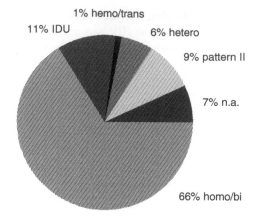

Figure 3.16 Distribution of AIDS cases in eastern Germany by means of transmission

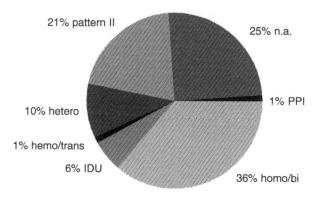

Figure 3.17 Means of transmission for newly-diagnosed people with HIV in eastern Germany, 1990–8

Germany has no immigration restrictions for people with HIV, except the state of Bavaria, where persons from non-EU countries who apply for a residency permit have to prove they are HIV-negative. Tests for HIV antibodies are also routinely performed in some states for persons who apply for political asylum in Germany. Although a positive test result has no effect on the decision about their application, it also does not automatically result in the provision of medical care. Officially, every person with legal residency status in Germany is entitled to social security benefits, including medical care, as required. If medical care, including anti-retroviral treatment, is necessary and treatment is not available in the country of origin, an argument can be made, based on humanitarian reasons, against imminent deportation. But since asylum seekers are in general not familiar with this prospect and they are sometimes not even informed about their test results, a considerable percentage of HIV-positive asylum seekers is deported upon rejection of their application. (See Deutsche AIDS-Hilfe, 1998).

Improved therapy and its effects on the epidemic

Since 1995-1996 the effectiveness of anti-retroviral therapy (ART) has been improved considerably by using triple or quadruple combination regimens. The broad publicity that accompanied these improvements led to a remarkable increase in the number of HIV-infected persons receiving ART, their number almost tripling between 1995 and 1999. The increasing efficacy of therapy and earlier initiation of treatment led to a significant decrease of AIDS-related deaths and AIDS-defining diseases. But the expectation that improved treatment would reduce the number of new infections has not yet materialised. As a consequence of a reduced death rate with no measurable change in the frequency of new infections, the actual number of people living with HIV/AIDS in Germany is currently increasing, after having been in a steady state since the early 1990s.

There is a number of reasons which might explain why the number of new infections is not declining, despite the fact that almost half of all people with HIV receive anti-retroviral treatment:

*   A large share of the ongoing HIV transmissions may result from unprotected intercourse between newly-infected, not-yet-diagnosed and therefore untreated HIV-positive persons and persons not yet infected.
*   A moderate decrease of infectivity of people under anti-retroviral therapy may be counteracted by an increase in risk behaviour.

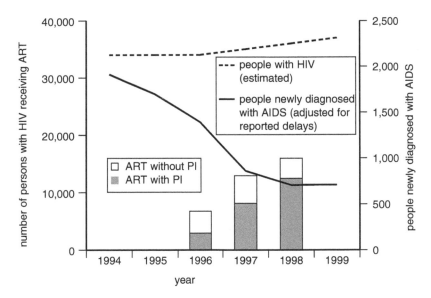

Figure 3.18 ART, AIDS incidence and HIV prevalence in Germany, 1995–9

- Possibly the decrease of infectivity of genital fluids under anti-retroviral therapy is smaller than suggested by the decrease of plasma viral load.

Conclusion

Among the larger Western industrialised countries, Germany is enjoying one of the lowest HIV prevalence and incidence rates. Only for the eastern part of the country can this be attributed to the delayed onset of the HIV epidemic. The western part of Germany became affected around the same time as the other Western European countries. Thus the remarkable success of the preventive efforts has to be explained either by unique characteristics of the most vulnerable groups or by specific features of the socio-political response.

Besides the demographically dispersed population of the gay community in Germany – which is comparable to Italy, Spain, and also to the US and Canada – there are hardly any obvious important differences between the gay communities in Germany and other Western European countries. In fact, the course of the HIV epidemic in the gay communities does not differ very much across Europe. There are, however, large differences between the HIV epidemics among the IV drug users, mainly between northern and southern European countries, which are not fully explained. Absolute size as well as the social settings of drug abuse and the socio-political attitudes to harm reduction approaches concerning drug abuse may play a role here. A specific German feature of the initial responses may be the early, pragmatic, and co-operative character of prevention campaigns in Germany which helped to avoid further marginalisation of people with HIV and ideological clashes between mainstream society and the primarily-affected groups. (See Frankenberg and Hannebeck, Chapter 4; Rosenbrock, Chapter 19; Rosenbrock *et al.*, Chapter 20.)

There is, however, a dark side to the prevention success. AIDS policy and the AIDS service movement fell into a 'prevention trap'. Though the actual epidemiology of HIV shows ongoing transmission on an unaltered scale, AIDS is increasingly becoming something which affects those without a voice in society. The largest group at risk as well as the group first infected with HIV – well-educated, middle class gay men – are being gradually replaced by lower class, less-educated gay men. The likely reason is that prevention has worked best for the middle class (Bochow, 1998).

The number of heterosexuals becoming infected through intercourse by partners without the traditional risk profiles is still so small that it seems more an accident-like event than one step further in a growing epidemic.

Perhaps because the epidemic is gradually losing the voice of the middle class, the public discourse on AIDS is becoming increasingly tedious and ritualised, with a tendency toward instrumentalising the issue for secondary purposes. Accompanying this development is a reduction in research funding, resulting in HIV research in Germany being reduced to a virtual invisibility and research capacities being redirected to other topics. Expenditures for prevention have been continuously reduced to the point where resources for piloting new and innovative approaches are no longer available. Consequently, the level of new infections could not be reduced any further during the last several years. (See Rosenbrock *et al.*, Chapter 20.)

One group that always has been neglected in prevention, prevention research and provision of care – the immigrant population, particularly men and women from developing countries – will continue to be neglected.

It could be argued that as long as the epidemic stays on the current level, AIDS does not justify any increased investment. This is, however, contingent on nothing changing, which is very unlikely. HIV epidemics continue to be quite unpredictable. The virus was present in countries like Russia, Ukraine, Thailand etc. years before epidemics began, and so far we have only partial explanations why the current epidemics started and what had delayed their onset. Accidental events play perhaps an important role. Even long-time stable epidemics can suddenly exacerbate due to seemingly minor changes in the conditions necessary for transmission. Among Vancouver's IV drug using population, for example, the incidence of HIV remained at a low level for several years before it suddenly soared. This was due to a shift in the consumption patterns from heroin to cocaine. With all other conditions being stable, the increase of injection frequencies may have been enough to alter the pattern of spread from low level endemic to an exponential increase of infections similar to a primary epidemic (Schechter *et al.*, 1999).

The continuing breakdown of the AIDS research and prevention infrastructure in Germany along with the declining quality of the public discourse on AIDS leaves the country in a vulnerable position should the epidemic alter its course. Euphoria in light of the positive results achieved by Germany in the first wave of the HIV/AIDS epidemic may well turn out to be premature, seriously handicapping the country in tackling a second wave, should it occur.

References

Bochow, M. (1998) 'Schichtspezifische Vulnerabilität im Hinblick auf HIV und AIDS', *Zeitschrift für Sexualforschung* 11: 327–45.

Connor, E. M., Sperling, R. S., Gelber, R. *et al.* (1994) 'Reduction of maternal-infant transmission of human immunodeficiency virus type 1 with zidovudine treatment', *New England Journal of Medicine* 331: 1173–80.

De Vincenzi, I., Jadand, C., Couturier, E. *et al.* (1997) 'Pregnancy and contraception in a French cohort of HIV-infected women', *AIDS* 11: 333–8.

Deutsche AIDS-Hilfe (1998) 'Handbuch Migration für AIDS-Hilfen', *AIDS-Fachkräfte und andere im AIDS-Bereich Tätige*, Berlin: Deutsche AIDS-Hilfe.

European Centre for the Epidemiological Monitoring of AIDS (quarterly reports) *HIV/AIDS Surveillance in Europe*.

Gerbase, A. C., Rowley, J. T., Heymann, D. H. L., Berkley, S. F. B. and Piot, P. (1998) 'Global prevalence and incidence estimates of selected curable STDs', *Sexual Transmission Information* 74 [Suppl. 1]: S12–16.

Hamers, F. (1996) 'AIDS associated with blood transfusion and haemophilia in Europe', *British Medical Journal* 312: 847–8.

Lutz-Friedrich, R. (1999) 'HIV und Schwangerschaft – Deutsche Zahlen', *Symposium Frauen und HIV*, Munich (April).

Markert, S. (1994) 'Risikoverhalten von Freiern', in W. Heckmann and M. A. Koch (eds), *Sexualverhalten in Zeiten von AIDS*, Berlin: edition sigma: 369–75.

Pauli, G., Vettermann, W., Marcus, U., Jovaisas, E. and Koch, M. A. (1985) 'Risikogruppen für AIDS', *Münchener medizinische Wochenschrift* 127: 42–5.

Schaefer, A., Koch, M.A., Grosch-Woerner, I. *et al.* (1994) 'Wehen, Geburtsmodus und maternofetale Transmission von HIV', *Geburtshilfe und Frauenheilkunde* 54: 617–22.

Schechter, M. T., Strathdee, S. A., Cornelisse, P. G. A., Currie, S., Patrick, D. M., Rekart, M. L. and O'Shaughnessy, M. V. (1999) 'Do needle exchange programmes increase the spread of HIV among injection drug users?: an investigation of the Vancouver outbreak', *AIDS* 13: F45–51.

Stephenson, J. M., Griffioen, A. *et al.* (1996) 'The effect of HIV diagnosis on reproductive experience',. *AIDS* 10: 1683-7.

Velten, D. and Kleiber, D (1994) 'HIV-Infektionsrisiken im Rahmen gewerblicher Sexualität: Zur Rolle der Freier', in W. Heckmann and M. A. Koch (eds), *Sexualverhalten in Zeiten von AIDS,* Berlin: edition sigma: 351–67.

4   From hysteria to banality

An overview of the political response to AIDS in Germany

Günter Frankenberg and Alexander Hanebeck

AIDS comes to Germany

The first press release from the German government naming AIDS as a national problem was issued in 1983.[1] Up to that point it was considered an American disease and therefore not a German issue. Soon after the press release a task force from San Francisco was invited by the Federal Ministry for Health to deliver firsthand information from those with the most experience regarding AIDS and its prevention. This visit helped to convince ministry officials to adopt a liberal approach, de-emphasizing the traditional public health response to the dangers of infectious diseases; namely, the Federal Law on Communicable Diseases (*Bundesseuchengesetz*). A second source of outside expertise was consulted when German medical experts and representatives of the gay community were invited to a secret meeting in the ministry to discuss methods of AIDS prevention. The reliance on groups that do not usually have easy access to governmental agencies indicated that public health authorities did not know much about the subject.

Maximalists and minimalists

Once the German government and the population as a whole became aware that AIDS was a disease which had to be taken seriously, most official reactions were sympathetic with regard to those infected and displayed a determination to gather information and to avoid panic. Exceptions to this restrained response were found in the tabloid press and in the government of Bavaria. In October 1983 a group of medical experts concluded that no extraordinary measures would be necessary because of the limitation of the disease to certain groups. But a press release by the Federal Ministry for Health in November 1984 declared that a new and strict 'Act for the Control of Diseases Transmitted by Sexual Contact' was being seriously considered. This proposal drew strong criticism as it included, among other measures, mandatory medical examinations for potentially infected persons, contact tracing, and reporting the names of those who refused medical treatment. By 1986 AIDS was a deeply contentious issue, with increasingly heated controversies about how to react to the spread of the disease. The battle lines were drawn between two groups who fought each other with an almost religious fervour. On the one side were the minimalists, including most state ministers of health and the Federal Ministry for Health. On the other side were the maximalists, most prominently the Bavarian state government.

Minimalism is critical of traditional coercive public health instruments like the Federal Law on Communicable Diseases and consequently limits governmental controls and intervention. Hence it relies on the co-operation of those at risk and was supported by most of the medical profession and the organisations and representatives of the so-called risk groups, most notably the Deutsche AIDS Hilfe (the National German AIDS Organisation), a largely gay community-based group. In general the minimalists believe that the contexts within which HIV is typically transmitted lie beyond governmental control and therefore coercion would be ineffective. They prefer AIDS to be treated differently from other communicable diseases, arguing for specific AIDS legislation providing the legal basis and the money for non-coercive interventions like sex education and the distribution of condoms and sterile syringes. In general the Federal Ministry for Health has relied on interventions of this kind, giving preference to information and support for self-help groups over governmental control and legal sanctions. Nevertheless, the option of turning to more restrictive measures in the event that the minimalist strategy would prove to be ineffective remained a distinct possibility. This was used as a back-up argument against accusations of not being tough enough in fighting the spread of the disease.

In contrast to this strategy, maximalism relies heavily on governmental control and intervention, employing the traditional methods of protecting the public's health: mandatory testing, mass screening, mandatory reporting and notification, surveillance, regulation of sites where risk behaviour occurs, quarantine, and imprisonment. These measures aim to identify the origins of an epidemic and to interrupt directly the chains of infection. Maximalists insist on treating all communicable diseases alike and maintain that each individual's knowing his/her own HIV status is a prerequisite for responsible behaviour. Therefore, everyone belonging to a risk group has the duty to know whether he or she is infected. Furthermore, maximalists believe in the importance of legal sanctions for irresponsible behaviour, convinced that such deterrence is necessary to serve the goals of prevention. Thus, maximalist appeals for co-operation from those at risk invariably have a threatening undertone. Supporters of this view usually include elements of minimalism in their argument, especially information and counselling, claiming that these measures can be linked effectively to contain-and-control interventions. It is important to stress, however, that despite these minimalist ingredients, the maximalist approach generally favours coercion over education and co-operation.

Although the legal system did not play a large role regarding prevention, legal arguments were symbolically important in the discourse about AIDS prevention strategies. Maximalists emphasized the rights of healthy people to be protected from the threat of AIDS, while minimalists insisted on the protection of the rights of infected persons against discrimination and their right to have access to medical care (Frankenberg, 1992).

In 1990 the debate became less aggressive and the importance of AIDS on the public agenda dwindled steadily. A minimalist approach was gradually accepted, although some issues – especially how much the government should press individuals to be tested – remained contested (Deutscher Bundestag, 1990).[2] Reunification did not bring about any significant changes.

The disease made the headlines again in 1993 during the scandal about blood products contaminated with the virus, in the wake of which the Federal Minister for Health, Horst Seehofer, once more proposed mass screening.[3] This can be attributed to the fears rekindled by the scandal and to the fact that two important elections were coming up in Bavaria, the state in which the maximalist approach was most popular and where Seehofer's party was trying to keep its comfortable majority. Interestingly, the same Minister proclaimed in 1997 that the Federal Government's approach had been a success, an approach which was in effect almost exclusively minimalist.[4] With the national election in 1998, the Social Democrats and the Greens took over the government. Since both of these parties have been strong proponents of a minimalist approach, the political climate is not likely to change.

AIDS in the public imagination

AIDS embodies mystery, sexuality and danger, making the disease a natural topic for the media. Before 1982 few articles were published; from 1983 on, coverage was intensive and continuous. Initially AIDS appeared in the media as an American problem; most of the articles were reports from the United States.[5] Once it could be presented as a threat for the 'normal' heterosexual population, and not just for marginalised groups, AIDS became a topic of primary interest (Ruehmann, 1985). The tabloids ran sensational human interest stories, for example, the story of the first infected German child or the drama of the 'infected nun'. The focus was, of course, on the still mysterious nature of the disease and even more on the sexual habits and appetites of promiscuous homosexuals, sometimes suggesting that the disease was the punishment for their sexual behaviour. Even the more highly respected newspapers and magazines were not void of homophobic slurs. In these publications the emphasis was on the biological and medical questions of HIV infection, satisfying the widespread public demand for information about the disease while debating how the further spread of AIDS could be avoided (Frankenberg, 1992).

The uncertainty about how HIV is transmitted led to articles claiming that the virus can fly through the air, and to reports of fear because an HIV infected person travelled on the same bus (Beule, 1999). Fear of AIDS was heightened by calculations predicting an explosive spread of the disease based on the assumption that the number of infected persons would double every year or even every six months (Beule, 1999). Some of the fears seem strange or even laughable today, now that we know exactly how the virus is transmitted. However, the uncertainties and the sensational reports by segments of the media had serious consequences for those infected. To a lesser extent these reports also had consequences for those belonging to groups with a high risk of infection, particularly homosexuals, because the associated fear led to discrimination (see below).

The German publication with the most extensive coverage of AIDS has always been *Der Spiegel*, a very influential weekly news magazine and a prime example of the changes in the way AIDS has been depicted in the media.[6] In 1983 AIDS was called a deadly *Seuche* on the cover, a word that translates as plague or scourge. In addition, the disease was closely linked to homosexuality by describing it as the 'homo-epidemic' or 'gay cancer' (*Der Spiegel*, 1983). A cover story in 1985 likened AIDS to the 'great plagues', among others the Black Death and cholera (*Der Spiegel*, 1985). From early on there were other accounts, interspersed with the apocalyptic stories, euphorically claiming that a cure is just around the corner. As early as 1986 the virus was declared to be 'decoded' (*Der Spiegel*, 1986) while in 1988 the magazine focused on the threat to everyone presented by the epidemic when it asked: 'AIDS – Couples in Danger?' (*Der Spiegel*, 1988). The optimistic articles began to dominate in the early 1990s, cumulating in a cover story announcing 'The AIDS Miracle' in 1997 (*Der Spiegel*, 1997).

These two angles on reporting about AIDS had different impacts. On the one hand, the basis for the currently widespread solidarity with HIV infected persons was cultivated by AIDS being depicted as an apocalyptic danger for everyone, not just for homosexuals. Groups like the AIDS service organisations (AIDS-Hilfen), who work with HIV patients and try to educate the public about the dangers of unprotected sex, won a high level of social prestige. In the last few years the President of Germany has been a sponsor of World AIDS Day. The red ribbon became a well-known symbol worn by many, including public figures, movie and television stars, talk show hosts and so on.

On the other hand, the optimistic descriptions about finding a cure and how successful infected persons have been treated, has trivialised the threat, leading to negative effects on prevention (Beule, 1999). Surveys by the Federal Centre for Health Education (*Bundeszentrale für gesundheitliche Aufklärung, BZgA*) show that AIDS awareness has been declining recently. AIDS is now seemingly depicted as being less dangerous, less lethal. There are new therapies resulting in HIV-infected persons surviving much longer than in the late 1980s. The quality of life for AIDS patients has increased dramatically, and the link between AIDS and death does not seem to be as inevitable as before (Dannecker, 1999). A patient at the University Hospital AIDS Centre in Frankfurt described his view of the future as 'normal – including the knowledge that it will be over at some point' (Bruns, 1999: 47). In the media *Langzeitüberlebende* (long-term survivors) has become a common term, making AIDS less unique, because it is no longer untreatable. In addition, new medical procedures give HIV-infected persons options they did not have a few years ago. For example, it is now possible to remove the virus from semen for artificial insemination. In Germany so far thirteen children have been born as a result of this new procedure, and none of the children or the mothers contracted HIV (Wessel, 1999). With such stories about how HIV-infected persons regain choices so they can lead almost 'normal' lives, AIDS is becoming less threatening and less unique. On World AIDS Day in the last few years one of the main topics has been the situation outside the industrialised world, where AIDS is rampant and the new therapies are not affordable. This situation is contrasted with that in Germany, where the AIDS epidemic is not perceived as being as serious any more.

The politics of public health

In its 1987 Emergency Programme to Fight AIDS the Federal Ministry for Health defined the three elements of its approach: protecting the population against infection, counselling and care for those infected, and preventing discrimination (Frankenberg, 1988a). The guiding principle was to give education and information precedence over traditional epidemiological control. This included measures authorised by the Federal Law on Communicable Diseases, which served as a backup and were to be used only in the case of 'incorrigible' individuals who recklessly put others at risk. The principal slogan was 'AIDS Concerns Everyone' (*AIDS geht alle an*), an attempt to overcome the perception that AIDS is just a problem for certain groups.

Peter Gauweiler, then Bavarian Secretary for Internal Affairs, was the driving force behind a campaign against this approach. The Bavarian government demanded stricter measures such as mandatory testing for soldiers and civil servants. Reaffirming its conservative profile, the Christian Social Union (CSU), the party in power in Bavaria, embedded this campaign in a moral crusade against 'national decadence' aimed at 'thinning out' sexually deviant groups. However, the Federal Ministry for Health, supported by the Conference of State Ministers of Health (see Frankenberg, 1988a) and the opposition parties (the Social Democrats and the Greens), isolated Bavaria. As a result, the Bavarian government issued its own catalogue of maximalist measures (Frankenberg, 1988a). However, a large part of these measures were merely proposals since the Bavarian government lacked the legal authority to implement them on its own. What they could do was regulate meeting places of at-risk groups; require the testing of persons suspected of being contagious; and implement mandatory testing for Bavarian civil servants, foreigners applying for residency permits, and prison inmates. The language of the recommended measures was aggressive, promoting testing as a crucial element in the control of AIDS. The legal duties of those infected and of those suspected of being infected as well as the punishment for non-compliance with these duties were at the core of the measures. As a result, the co-operation of those most at-risk was stifled in that part of the country.

In contrast, the Federal Government and all other state governments implemented a non-aggressive program opposing mandatory measures and seeking the co-operation of those most affected by AIDS. Voluntary testing was recommended. The program relied heavily on information campaigns by the Federal Centre for Health Education (BZgA) which began to inform the general population about AIDS in 1985. (See Pott, Chapter 6.) Considerable funds for these campaigns were allocated from 1987 on. Over the years the campaigns have used ads in magazines as well as television and cinema advertisements, posters, and brochures aimed at the wider public. The various campaigns also seek to inform professionals who have direct contact with the target groups (for example, social workers, teachers, medical professionals). The messages focus not only on providing the necessary information about how the virus is transmitted and how to prevent infection but also how to overcome irrational fears while enhancing solidarity with HIV infected persons. In addition, federal funds were used to support AIDS service organisations and local public health departments. This included funding to hire an AIDS specialist for each of the 309 public health departments so as to professionalise the counselling, the outreach work, and school-based sex education related to AIDS (see Miesala-Edel and Schöps-Potthoff, Chapter 5).[7]

Over the years the official message shifted from 'AIDS Concerns Everyone' to 'Don't Give AIDS a Chance'. Because of advances in therapies leading to the recognition that early clinical intervention can be critical, anonymous HIV counselling and testing has been given greater emphasis.

The threat of HIV infection clearly revealed the inadequacies of the official drug policy.[8] Traditionally all anti-drug measures had to have abstinence as their goal. Alternative programs, such as methadone maintenance, were either illegal or considered to be counterproductive. Policy was guided by the belief that coercion and criminalisation were necessary as an external motivation for a successful therapy. This approach resulted in only 20 per cent of drug users seeking counselling and less than 6 per cent seeking inpatient treatment, most of them unsuccessfully (Kreuzer, 1990; Rosenbrock, 1986; Barsch, Chapter 14). Until the mid-1980s drug counsellors were unsure about the legality of dispensing disposable needles, and many viewed the distribution of needles and syringes as promoting addiction.

This attitude began to change in 1983 when sterile needles were made available in various parts of the country (except in Bavaria and in its neighbouring state of Baden-Württemberg). More problematic was the introduction of methadone programs, which was opposed by the medical profession and drug counsellors alike, who saw drug use primarily as a social – not as a medical – problem. With HIV spreading rapidly, especially among intravenous drug users, this position weakened. In March 1987 the public health ministers of all states except Bavaria proposed that methadone treatment was justifiable in special cases and under strict medical supervision. Shortly thereafter the Federal Government approved methadone treatment in individual cases where there was medical cause. In 1990 the changing attitude in the medical profession became apparent when the federal Medical Council (*Bundesgesundheitsamt*) declared the provision of methadone acceptable.

German drug policy has thus been modifed by AIDS, from the idea of a drug-free life as a precondition for public assistance toward outreach services for long-term drug users. The government of Bavaria is still the most visible opponent of such an approach. However, in the platform of the new coalition government elected in October 1998, the Social Democrats and the Greens declared that they want to strengthen the outreach programs in some larger cities.[9] In addition, they want to follow the lead of some state governments which are offering drug-substitution programs, based on models in Switzerland. These programs provide long-term drug users not only with methadone but also – under physician supervision and close scientific scrutiny – with the drugs they are addicted to, like heroin. (For a discussion of the new approaches to drug treatment in Germany, see Barsch, Chapter 14.)

The limited reaction of the public health system to AIDS generated a number of non-governmental responses, the most important and influential being the Deutsche AIDS-Hilfe and its members at the local level, a network of self-help groups unique in the German public health context. (See Schillling, Chapter 8 and Etgeton, Chapter 7.)

AIDS and the law

During the period of heated discussion about the best AIDS prevention strategy, the approach of the Federal Government was challenged in the Federal Constitutional Court. The complainant, a haemophiliac, argued that the Government was not doing enough to protect him against AIDS and called for legislative measures. In its dismissal of the case the Court insisted that the Federal Government had neither remained inactive nor acted ineffectively, thereby implicitly rejecting the claim that AIDS must be treated like other sexually transmitted diseases. This ruling allowed for a distinctive approach toward AIDS, strengthening the position of minimalists (Bundesverfassungs-gericht, 1987). No cases came before the lower courts regarding prevention policy.[10]

Discrimination has been a very real problem for HIV-infected persons in Germany, despite the information campaigns of the Federal Centre for Health Education. The widespread knowledge that HIV is not easily transmitted notwithstanding, AIDS has evoked panic reactions. More often than not, the spirit of solidarity extolled in public statements quickly vanished behind irrational fears of contagion. Employees have demanded that an infected co-worker be fired, threatening to quit themselves if their demands were not met. Physicians and dentists have refused to treat those suspected of having AIDS, and landlords have sought to evict persons with AIDS from their apartments. (See Frankenberg, 1988b, for further examples.) Because of the stigma and discrimination even AIDS activists have been at times unable to reveal their HIV-positive status to families and friends, causing some to pretend that they have a different disease, like pneumonia or leukaemia.

Although discrimination has decreased, it has continued to be a problem. In spite of this, no anti-discrimination statute has been formally proposed, probably because instances of discrimination have not led to many cases of flagrant exclusion practices in the workplace.[11] Another reason could be that no consensus could be reached among supporters about the proper form for such legislation, as Germany has no tradition of anti-discrimination laws protecting specific groups.

This situation may change since the new government elected in the autumn of 1998 announced that a comprehensive anti-discrimination act is one of the goals they want to achieve. However, the announcement does not contain any reference to AIDS and so far no specific proposals have been put forward.

In the absence of such a law, the right to privacy (in German law: *Allgemeines Persönlichkeitsrecht, Art. 2 I* and *1 I Grundgesetz*) and the right to 'self-determination over personal information', entitle every individual to have control over the disclosure and use of information about one's self. This right has won great significance in recent years. Originally created by legal scholars and only officially recognised in 1983 by the Federal Constitutional Court (Bundesverfassungsgericht, 1983), the right to privacy regarding personal information can only be questioned in the case of a compelling public interest. In the context of the debates about AIDS, this opinion has strengthened the minimalist position, helping to defeat proposals for mandatory testing and reporting and plans for HIV testing without consent in hospitals.

Besides the significant role it has played in the political debate about AIDS, the right to privacy has helped to protect the rights of individuals in court. While in 1989 a local court (Amtsgericht Mölln, 1989) ruled that there was no violation of rights in conducting an HIV test without consent, a recent decision of a district court expressed an opposing view. In that case a dermatologist was sued for damages because he had conducted an HIV test without the consent of the patient, a homosexual who had deliberately chosen not to be tested and who practised safer sex. According to the patient, the dermatologist had argued that the test was necessary in order to protect himself and his staff. In court, the dermatologist's defence rested on the claim that the patient, by consenting to a medical examination, implicitly consented to the HIV test. The district court in Cologne held that such a test without prior consent of the patient is a grave violation of the right to privacy, whether the test is deemed medically necessary or not. The patient was awarded 1,500 marks in damages (Landgericht Köln, 1995). Since the legal consequences of HIV tests without the prior consent of the patient are not entirely clear, legal scholars advise physicians not to conduct any tests without the patient's consent.[12] Implicit consent is regarded as sufficient only if the patient has symptoms which indicate that she or he is suffering from AIDS (Uhlenbruck, 1996).

The blood product scandal

In 1993 a scandal broke that led to a parliamentary committee of inquiry and the dissolution of the federal agency overseeing pharmaceutical products. The tragedy behind the scandal is that almost 50 per cent of haemophiliacs were infected if treated with blood products before these products became subject to mandatory HIV tests. Since October 1985 the test has been mandatory for all new products, though those already in circulation were not recalled. The testing proved to be effective, so that by 1994 no new infections caused by blood transfusions or the use of blood products were reported. The events causing this tragedy have been likened to the Contergan/Thalidomide case, making it the second post-war catastrophe in the pharmaceutical industry (Hart, 1995).

Early in 1987, before the tragedy became a scandal, the pharmaceutical industry and their insurance companies began to negotiate with groups representing haemophiliacs to settle claims for damages out of court. The negotiating position of the haemophiliacs was weak for three reasons. First, it was technically a difficult case, as most haemophiliacs had been treated with products from different companies, making it almost impossible to establish causality between the product of one company and a specific infection (Deutscher Bundestag, 1994). Second, trying to put public pressure on the pharmaceutical industry was not an option because the vast majority of infected haemophiliacs did not want publicity for fear of being stigmatised once the infection became known. In the mid to late 1980s AIDS was still widely associated with promiscuity, homosexuality, prostitution and drug use. Many believed anonymity was the only option to avoid social isolation. The final report of the parliamentary committee of inquiry reports a case in which the widow of a haemophiliac asked a nationwide support group for haemophiliacs not to send a wreath to the funeral, although her husband had been a leading member of the group. She feared isolation in the rural community she lived in, where nobody had known about her husband's disease. The third reason the haemophiliacs case was weak had to do with the time pressure for the HIV-infected persons. Because of their short life expectancy they simply could not wait much longer. Under these circumstances most haemophiliacs saw no choice other than to accept the settlement, although they felt the negotiations had been conducted in a humiliating fashion and found the result to be inadequate (Deutscher Bundestag, 1994).

The parliamentary committee of inquiry was triggered by the public debate concerning the role of the Federal Ministry for Health with regard to the HIV contaminated blood products. Hysteria reared its ugly head again in the media with headlines like 'Death by Prescription' or 'Deadly Blood', with reports stating that 'thousands were given deadly injections'. In its final report the committee concluded that the pharmaceutical industry, medical professionals, hospitals, and the bodies legally and economically responsible for them – including the Ministry – had a joint legal responsibility for the infection of haemophiliacs after 1983. Approximately 60 per cent of the infections could have been avoided (Deutscher Bundestag, 1994). To what degree the committee viewed each player to be responsible can be seen by looking at the proposal for a fund to compensate the victims. The pharmaceutical industry and its insurance companies were expected to carry 60 per cent of the financial burden, the states 15 per cent, the Federal Government 20 per cent, and the medical profession 5 per cent (Deutscher Bundestag, 1994).

Compensation remained one of the most contested issues. During the parliamentary debate about the final report of the inquiry committee Horst Seehofer, the Federal Minister for Health, apologised to the victims in the name of the Government for the mistakes that were made. Furthermore, he announced that a fund would be established with assets of almost 700 million marks, out of which the damages for the victims would be paid. As the inquiry committee had suggested, 60 per cent of the money should come from the pharmaceutical industry. The fund that finally resulted from negotiations with the parties involved had assets worth only 250 million marks, the biggest share being paid by the Federal Government. Every HIV-infected person was to receive monthly payments of 1,500 marks, every person suffering from AIDS 3,000, and children and partners of victims 1,000. Whoever accepted the pension forfeited the option to sue any of the parties contributing to the fund for damages.[13] According to the first paragraph of the act, the fund is to provide 'humanitarian' and 'social' aid, which is a far cry from the legal (co-)responsibility described by the inquiry committee. The pharmaceutical industry insisted that their giving money to the fund was not an admission of any responsibility or guilt. This 'humanitarian' solution infuriated the victims for several reasons. They felt betrayed, especially because the fund's assets were much smaller than announced earlier in the year. In addition, a monthly payment was not seen as adequate compensation, given that most of the victims had been infected more than ten years prior and their life expectancy was short.

AIDS loses its special status

The debate about AIDS prevention was effectively put to rest in favour of minimalism and a pragmatic strategy, without achieving unanimity in the country. No longer inevitably associated with death, AIDS is losing what made it fundamentally different from other epidemics. There are now seldom horror stories in the media; it is the therapeutic advances which dominate reports about AIDS. Because of this, a process of normalisation has set in. This does not mean that AIDS suddenly became harmless or is being treated as if it were so, but it has lost its exceptionalism. Therefore new problems are being faced by HIV-infected persons, groups like the AIDS service organisations and others involved in AIDS prevention and care. (See Rosenbrock *et al.*, Chapter 20.)

One of the issues is funding. Public budgets are tight and public spending has been cut in many areas, including support for AIDS prevention and self help groups. For example, the AIDS prevention budget of the Federal Centre for Health Education was cut by a third in 1997. The Deutsche AIDS-Hilfe, the National German AIDS Organisation, lost all public funding for their office of public relations, resulting in the cancellation of their quarterly magazine which was distributed free of charge in places like schools and hospitals.

The social and financial situation for people with HIV is also no longer exceptional, though still marked by serious difficulties. Social security, especially health insurance, has been modified in the last few years. Though new regulations were not aimed at HIV-infected persons specifically, they have had serious effects on this group. Patients now have to pay a larger share out of their own pocket, which affects HIV-infected persons and everyone else in need of long-term treatment more than it affects the average patient. Court battles are not touching on the big issues anymore, but deal rather with the smaller problems of daily life with HIV. For example, the Federal Administrative Court held that, under certain circumstances, a homosexual on public welfare has to be given additional money to be able to buy condoms as a form of preventive health care (Bundesverwaltungsgericht, 1995).

Not only the religious fervour of the debate about AIDS has abated, but AIDS in general has lost its position as an issue of special interest on the political agenda. How much AIDS has been out of the public eye can best be illustrated by the federal election campaigns in 1998. The term AIDS or HIV did not appear in the platform of any major party, including the Greens, who have been the most responsive to the demands of self-help groups and for whom equal rights for homosexuals is still an issue.

AIDS has lost its uniqueness for Germany; it is but one issue among others competing for public attention and money. It went from being the mother of all epidemics, instilling widespread fear, to becoming one of the many serious risks one has to deal with in modern life. AIDS went from being *the* epidemic of the twentieth century to becoming just another epidemic.

Notes

1 The article is based in part on Frankenberg, G. (1992) 'Germany: the uneasy triumph of pragmatism', in D. Kirp and R. Bayer (eds), *AIDS in the Industrialized Democracies*, New Brunswick, N.J.: Rutgers University Press: 99–133.
2 It was agreed upon that the most important and effective weapon against the spread of AIDS is education and counselling, but no consensus could be reached concerning the use of coercive measures in individual cases. (See Deutscher Bundestag, 1990: 186.)
3 For an account of the scandal see the report of the parliamentary inquiry committee (Deutscher Bundestag, 1994).
4 As noted above, the option of turning to more restrictive measures was kept in reserve but never actually implemented.
5 For example, AIDS was called the 'evil that comes from America'; for more examples see Frankenberg (1992).
6 *Der Spiegel* has run twenty cover stories on AIDS since 1983.
7 For a comprehensive description of government activities concerning AIDS prevention see Deutscher Bundestag, 1990: 262–281.
8 The discussion here focuses on HIV and drug users. For information about the target group prostitutes, see Frankenberg, 1992: 106ff.
9 The most innovative projects exist in Frankfurt and Hamburg, the cities with the largest group of drug addicts in Germany, apart from Berlin.
10 Lower courts did, however, write opinions which discuss the issues in the debate between maximalism and minimalism. For examples see Frankenberg, 1992: 126–8.
11 There are some regulations that protect HIV-infected persons from exclusion in the workplace. HIV tests for prospective employees and questions about HIV infections by the employer are only admissible if the employer has a legitimate interest in the information, for example, in the case of nurses and doctors. An employee can not be fired because he/she is seropositive. Only if a person becomes too sick to work can he/she be dismissed under the same regulations applying to employees with other long-term illnesses. (See Laufs and Reiling, 1995).
12 The contradictions in the court rulings with regard to damages for HIV tests without consent is only one example of the still unclear situation in many areas of law related to HIV where no federal court has ruled on the issue. For more examples see

Frankenberg, 1992. For a short but comprehensive overview of AIDS-related questions in different legal areas see Laufs and Reiling, 1995.

13   For a more detailed description of the act establishing the fund see Deutsch, 1996.

References

Amtsgericht Mölln (1989) 'Urteil vom 6. 10. 1988', *Neue Juristische Wochenschrift* 12: 775.

Beule, J. (1999) '*Zwischen Apokalypse und Euphorie*' (Between apocalypse and euphoria), *Forschung Frankfurt* vol. 1: 54ff.

Bruns, I. (1999) 'Ich bin zwar positiv, aber ich denke positiv' (I am indeed positive, but I still think positive), *Forschung Frankfurt* 1: 44ff.

Bundesverfassungsgericht (Federal Constitutional Court) (1983) *Entscheidungen des Bundesverfassungsgerichts* (Decisions of the Federal Constitutional Court) 65, 1.

—— (1987), in *Neue Juristische Wochenschrift* 37: 2287–8.

Bundesverwaltungsgericht (Federal Administrative Court) (1995) *Familienrechtszeitung* 10: 599.

Dannecker, M. (1999) 'AIDS – eine ganz normale Krankheit?' (AIDS – just your ordinary disease?), *Forschung Frankfurt* 1: 48–52.

Deutsch, E. (1996) 'Das Gesetz über die humanitäre Hilfe für durch Blutprodukte HIV-Infizierte' (The Act concerning humanitarian help for persons infected through blood products), *Neue Juristische Wochenschrift* 12: 755–8.

Deutscher Bundestag (1990) 'Abschlußbericht der Enquete-Kommission des Deutschen Bundestages 'Gefahren von AIDS und wirksame Wege zu ihrer Eindämmung, AIDS: Fakten und Konsequenzen" (Final peport of the Enquete Commission of the Federal Parliament: 'The dangers of AIDS and effective measures for its containment'), *Bundestagsdrucksache* 11/7200, Bonn: Deutscher Bundestag.

—— (1994) 'Abschlußbericht des Untersuchugsausschusses 'HIV-Infektionen durch Blut und Blutprodukte" (Final Report of Parliamentary Inquiry Committee on HIV-Infections caused by Blood or Blood-Products), *Bundestagsdrucksache* 12/8591, Bonn: Deutscher Bundestag.

Frankenberg, G. (1988a) 'AIDS-Bekämpfung im Rechtsstaat, Aufklärung – Zwang – Prävention' (AIDS-Control and the Rule of Law, Education – Coercion – Prevention), Baden Baden: Nomos Verlagsgesellschaft.

—— (1988b) 'Innere Sicherheit in Zeiten der Infektion?' (Law and order in light of contagion), in *Kritische Vierteljahresschrift für Gesetzgebung und Rechtswissenschaft* 4: 344–5.

—— (1992) 'Germany: the uneasy triumph of pragmatism', in D. Kirp and R. Bayer (eds), *AIDS in the Industrialized Democracies*, New Brunswick, N.J.: Rutgers University Press.

Hart, D. (1995) 'HIV-Infektionen durch Blut und Blutprodukte' (HIV infection through blood and blood products), *Medizinrecht* 2: 63ff.

Kreuzer, A. (1990) 'Besonderheiten von AIDS und Drogenabhängigkeit' (The special issues associated with AIDS and drug addiction), in C. Prittwitz (ed.), *AIDS, Recht und Gesundheitspolitik* (AIDS, the law and public health policy), Berlin: edition sigma: 171ff.

Landgericht Köln (1995) 'Urteil vom 8. 2. 1995', *Neue Juristische Wochenschrift* 24: 1621–2.

Laufs, A. and Reiling, E. (1995) 'Rechtsfragen zur HIV-Infektion und AIDS-Erkrankung', (Legal Questions concerning HIV infection and AIDS), Frankfurt/Main: pmi Verlagsgruppe.

Rosenbrock, R. (1986) 'AIDS kann schneller besiegt werden' (AIDS can be defeated more quickly), Hamburg: VSA Verlag.

Ruehmann, F. (1985) AIDS – Eine Krankheit und ihre Folge (AIDS – a disease and its consequences), Frankfurt/Main and New York: Campus Verlag: Chapter 2.

Der Spiegel (1983) 'Tödliche Seuche AIDS – Die rätselhafte Krankheit', 6 June: 23.

—— (1985) 'Die großen Seuchen – AIDS, Syphilis, Pest, Cholera, Pocken', 23 September: 39.

—— (1986) 'AIDS – Das enträtselte Virus', 28 April: 18.

—— (1988) 'AIDS – Paare in Gefahr?', 22 February: 8.

—— (1997) 'Ende des Sterbens – Das AIDS-Wunder', 3 January: 2.

Uhlenbruck, W. (1996) 'Schmerzensgeld wegen HIV-Test ohne Einwilligung des Patienten' (Damages for pain and suffering caused by HIV tests without the patient's consent), *Medizinrecht* vol. 5: 206ff.

Wessel, C. (1999) 'Dreizehn Versuche wider das Schicksal', *Süddeutsche Zeitung*, 21 April: 3.

5 The role of the German Federal Government in fighting the epidemic

Dorle Miesala-Edel and Martina Schöps-Potthoff

AIDS and the structure of the health care system in Germany

In 1987 the German Federal Government adopted an Emergency Programme to Fight AIDS. More than ten years later, the disease continues to be a serious problem; however, the dismal forecasts from the mid-1980s regarding the spread of HIV failed to materialise.

In Germany, AIDS met with a structurally and materially secure health care system made up of a multitude of governmental and non-governmental institutions that contribute to the health of the general public, both in terms of health promotion and curative care. Of particular importance are the statutory health insurance funds whose legal mandate it is to guarantee their members comprehensive coverage in the case of illness. They ensure that each patient receives the necessary medical treatment irrespective of their age, sex, or social class and independent of the type of disease. (See Wright, Chapter 2, for a description of health insurance in Germany.) In addition, a variety of charitable organisations contribute to the provision of health care. These include the Social Welfare Associations in particular (*Verbände der Freien Wohlfahrtspflege;* see Wright, Chapter 2.) In Germany, legislative power regarding health issues is shared between the Federal Government and the Länder (the sixteen federal states) as stipulated by Article 74 of the Basic Law in the German Constitution (Art. 74, *Grundgesetz*; see 'federalism' in Wright, Chapter 2).

The tasks of the health care system on the federal and Länder level are executed by various ministries and authorities. On the federal level, responsibility for issues relating to preventive health care and disease control – particularly the control of AIDS and other communicable diseases – lies directly with the Federal Ministry for Health. The Ministry receives scientific support in these matters from the Robert Koch Institute (RKI), a public authority directly subordinate to the Ministry. One of the RKI's primary tasks is to collect and evaluate national epidemiological data regarding HIV infections and AIDS cases. Since 1982, the RKI has kept the national AIDS case registry. (See Marcus, Chapter 3.)

The Federal Ministry for Health is also responsible for the activities of the

Federal Centre for Health Education (*Bundeszentrale für gesundheitliche Aufklärung – BZgA*) which is assigned the task of providing information about the infection risks and means of prevention for HIV and other diseases. The BZgA's prevention-oriented activities are generally addressed to the public at large and not to a specific segment of the population. (See Pott, Chapter 6.) The practical work of prevention at the grassroots level is done by the local public health offices.

Responsibility for the testing and licensing of commercial HIV tests lies with the Paul Ehrlich Institute (PEI), which is the body in Germany responsible for the approval and monitoring of vaccines, serological tests, and blood preparations.

A key role in co-ordinating the various activities nationally is played by the Conference of Health Ministers (*Gesundheitsministerkonferenz – GMK*) and the Federal Committee of Länder for the Co-ordination AIDS Education Programmes (*Bund-Länder Gremium zur Koordinierung von Maßnahmen der AIDS-Aufklärung*) which meets twice a year.

The non-governmental sector is also an important element in the overall prevention strategy. A particular advantage of non-governmental organisations, such as the regional AIDS service organisations (*AIDS-Hilfen*), is their proximity to specific target groups. In many cases, their counselling activities are funded by the Länder and local governments. Thanks to this funding, it has also been possible to improve the co-ordination and co-operation between individual institutions involved in AIDS prevention and care, effectively complementing the policies of the Federal Government. National co-ordination and technical support for the local and regional AIDS service organisations is provided by the Deutsche AIDS-Hilfe, the National Federation of German AIDS Service Organisations, which is funded by the Ministry for Health through moneys made available to the Federal Centre for Health Education (BZgA). (See Pott, Chapter 6; Schilling, Chapter 8.)

The situation in Germany in 1987: the foundation is laid

At the beginning of the epidemic media coverage alternated between hype and understatement, and the debate over the right approach to controlling the disease became very emotional. (See Frankenberg and Hanebeck, Chapter 4.) In 1987 dramatic extrapolations put the number of those infected at 80,000, a caseload we have not reached to this day, even with the substantial population increase due to unification. Moreover, by European and international standards, Germany ranks favourably regarding the number of individuals infected with HIV and the number of AIDS patients. (See Marcus, Chapter 3.) Back in 1987, however, the population at large was uneasy. At that time, the number of diagnosed AIDS cases in Germany totalled 290. As fear and insecurity mounted, the call for state intervention grew louder. Against this backdrop it is all the more significant that we managed to design a scientifically-based strategy of AIDS control using available epidemiological data which has proved to be the correct policy, even in retrospect.

With respect to the objectives of the national prevention strategy, there was near universal agreement on the following:

- Containment of the disease by preventing new infections.
- Development of effective medication and a vaccine as well as the promotion of clinical research, more generally.
- Provision of an optimal level of counselling and care for those affected, requiring the development of appropriate service structures.
- Creation of a climate of solidarity throughout the whole society for people with HIV/AIDS.

In 1987 the divergence in opinion mainly concerned the approach which should be taken in order to attain these goals. There were two basic points-of-view:

- Using disease control and containment measures as stipulated by the Federal Law on Communicable Diseases (*Bundesseuchengesetz*) which includes isolating those affected, if necessary.
- Combating the disease by means of education, motivational strategies, and counselling with the goal of strengthening a sense of personal responsibility.

The controversies were openly argued in the media, the debate eventually supporting the implementation of an education-based strategy. (See Frankenberg and Hanebeck, Chapter 4, for a description of this debate.) This approach rejected the use of coercion, instead trusting in people's ability to learn and to pursue voluntarily protective life-styles. The Emergency Programme to Fight AIDS was thus drafted on the basis of an agreement adopted by the Governing Coalition. Incidentally, the approach which was adopted was by no means original to Germany, but was designed to be in line with the WHO's health promotion principles and the recommendations of the European Commission. The strategies called for in the Emergency Programme were based not only on the specifics of the disease and its routes of transmission, but also on ideas of a 'proper' management of the disease which were guided by ethical considerations.

The German parliament, the Bundestag, also instituted an Enquete Commission to deliberate on the most effective means for controlling the spread of HIV. The Commission included nine Members of Parliament from all four parties represented in the Bundestag and eight experts from various disciplines. In its final report submitted in 1990, the Commission endorsed the goals and implementation strategy outlined in the Emergency Programme. In their judgement, the programme represented 'a concept of modern public health policy in keeping with current knowledge and the available resources, devised to address an emerging disease that is predominantly transmitted by sexual contacts and drug use' (Deutscher Bundestag, 1990: 492). Many of the policies and projects launched over the years in fighting the epidemic stemmed from suggestions which evolved in the course of the Commission's work.

In addition to the above, the National AIDS Advisory Committee (*Nationaler*

AIDS Beirat) was appointed in 1987 as an independent panel of experts from the fields of medicine, nursing, social work, psychology, the sexual sciences, the social insurance bodies, etc. An AIDS Co-ordination Unit (*AIDS Koordinationsstelle*) was also set up in what was then the Federal Ministry for Youth, Family Affairs, Women and Health and funds for AIDS prevention and various pilot projects were earmarked in the federal budget for a four-year period.[1] Finally, the Ordinance on the Reporting of Laboratory Results (*Laborberichtsverordnung*) was implemented nationwide, requiring each laboratory to report positive HIV test results anonymously to the Robert Koch Institute in Berlin. Also, the Conference of Health Ministers (GMK), in which the Federal and Länder governments work closely together, adopted important resolutions at this time which reflected their universally agreed upon position.

From the outset, the Federal Government also co-operated with non-governmental organisations in combating the immunodeficiency disease. The most important partner in the self-help sector continues to be the Deutsche AIDS-Hilfe (DAH), as mentioned earlier. The DAH, a recognised charity in the health field, is made up of persons with HIV/AIDS, members of the groups primarily affected by AIDS, their partners, friends and families, as well as committed members from the general public. Founded in 1983, the Berlin-based parent association meanwhile has a membership of about 120 local AIDS service organisations. Thus the DAH now has a comprehensive self-help network in both the former West and East Germany, with several thousand volunteers and about 400 full-time staff. (See Schilling, Chapter 8; Etgeton, Chapter 7.) Among the most important tasks of the DAH and its members are planning and implementing nation-wide information and prevention campaigns as well as the development, production, and dissemination of target group-specific information material. The Federal Government leaves it to the discretion of the DAH to judge whether or not a given measure is appropriate for the target group intended. The parent association is largely financed by the Federal Centre for Health Education (BZgA) with funds from the Federal Ministry for Health. Whereas in 1987 the DAH received approximately 4.6 million marks for its work, funding in subsequent years has ranged between 5.9 and 7.4 million.

From the beginning there has been an explicitly agreed upon sharing of tasks between governmental and non-governmental institutions. The DAH, being an association of self-help groups, focuses on the needs of specific target populations, particularly on the needs of homosexual men and other primarily affected groups. The Federal Government, in contrast, mainly focuses its prevention activities on the general public and certain segments of the population, such as young persons, through the activities of the Federal Centre for Health Education. This task-sharing has proved successful, resulting in campaigns with a high level of authenticity and credibility for the populations targeted. (See also Pott, Chapter 6.)

Another important institution established in 1987 at the suggestion of the Federal Chancellor at the time, Helmut Kohl, was the National AIDS Foundation. In 1996 it joined forces with *Positiv leben*, another AIDS foundation also set up in 1987, to become the German AIDS Foundation (*Deutsche AIDS-Stiftung – DAS*), a non-profit organisation based in Bonn. The German AIDS Foundation is committed to addressing acute emergencies by providing people with HIV/AIDS with direct financial assistance for specific needs. Most applicants for assistance are young people, as this age group only rarely has private insurance or other means for securing their livelihood, and they frequently have not yet contributed enough to the national pension plan in order to make a claim. As a result, many young people with HIV/AIDS have to live on social assistance. In cases where this benefit does not adequately cover the costs of the disease, the Foundation steps in, providing fast, non-bureaucratic help. In addition to individual grants, the Foundation also envisages funding projects for the care and support of HIV-infected persons and AIDS patients. The Foundation can also support research projects, but this kind of funding is rare. Not only did the Federal Government donate 4 million marks to the Foundation, but it has been actively supporting its work through fund-raising campaigns. The Federal Minister for Health is a member of the Foundation's board of directors.

Special initiatives of the Federal Government to fight AIDS: education, pilot projects and research

Implementation of the Emergency Programme to Fight AIDS was made possible thanks to the deployment of substantial funds. Up to now, the Federal Government alone has invested more than 717 million marks in AIDS control, approximately 336 million for education, approximately 232 million for pilot projects and approximately 109 million for research and development projects. A total of 40 million marks was made available as a subsidy toward the support of persons injured through HIV-infected blood and blood products. (See below and also Frankenberg and Hanebeck, Chapter 4.) Moreover, from the beginning of the epidemic until 1998, a total of approximately 68 million marks, earmarked for education campaigns, funded projects of the Deutsche AIDS-Hilfe. In 1999, the DAH was to receive 6.8 million.

Education

From the beginning, the Federal Government has felt committed to an effective prevention strategy based on information, voluntary participation, and behaviour change. It must be borne in mind that the Government had hardly any experience when it came to preventing a disease which touched on social taboos such as death and sex. At the same time, however, the Government had to defend and guarantee the civil rights of those affected. This was what made the development of a control strategy so difficult. Eventually, the pillars of prevention came to be education, counselling, the rational and considered use of the HIV test, and the employment of personal protective behaviours. The national campaign has succeeded in effectively removing taboos from condom use. (See Pott, Chapter 6.)

Pilot projects as instruments in AIDS prevention policy

In Germany, pilot projects have been important instruments of innovative policy-making since the mid-1960s. First and foremost, they serve as 'field trials' for social and health policy, preceding the launch of reform measures. They are mostly created to address tasks which cannot be executed on a large scale owing to a lack of know-how and experience or to deficits and shortcomings in the existing array of services. Pilot projects, which can be individual initiatives as well as large-scale programmes, can be initiated by a federal ministry. The projects are proposed and implemented by both governmental institutions and voluntary associations, including self-help organisations and other entities responsible for social and health policy.

The Federal Government's power to fund projects in political areas in which it has no explicit administrative responsibility was no longer controversial by the time AIDS emerged. An important decision by the Federal Constitutional Court (*Bundesverfassungsgericht*) ruled that pilot projects may not *de facto* take the form of on-going federal budget items but must be restricted to a time-limited support of efforts designed to gather knowledge and test hypotheses in a given area. Another condition is that the pilot projects be of legislative importance or that they realise tasks incumbent on the sponsoring ministry.

With regard to AIDS, new methods and concepts for counselling, care, and support had to be developed and tested, and services already in place needed review and improvement. These tasks had to be accomplished within the framework of the Emergency Programme to Fight AIDS launched in 1987. Technically and professionally the pilot projects helped to gather experience and to support and advance new developments. At the same time, they were designed in such a way as to explore the legal, organisational, and financial issues raised. Each of the pilot projects launched had a specific task and goal, for example:

Health department expansion In order to support their AIDS control programmes, all of the 309 local public health offices in the then West Germany were provided with the funding to employ one AIDS specialist each (a doctor, psychologist, or social worker). The target population took extensive advantage of the counselling offered by the AIDS specialists: within three months, pilot project staff carried out 32,000 face-to-face and 20,000 telephone counselling sessions in the health department offices. They staged approxi-mately 2,200 educational events in school classes, with teachers, and with parents, and provided advice in over 2,500 health care facilities and social insurance institutions, as well as in companies and voluntary associations. (See Thoben *et al.*, 1991.)

AIDS-related psychosocial counselling This pilot project dealt with coun-selling in special conflict situations in particular, and with the development of counselling standards in general. A staff of approximately thirty members was assembled to help their clients in coping with psychological and social problems related to AIDS. They provided in-depth counselling to HIV-positive persons and to others seeking advice regarding several issues; for example, the HIV antibody test, specific lifestyles, coping with current crises, and dealing with public authorities. (See Filsinger *et al.*, 1993.)

Outreach work   Chiefly employed by public health departments and AIDS service organisations, forty-six outreach workers were active in twenty-six cities in Germany. Their goal was to promote and consolidate AIDS preventive behaviour in the most affected groups via outreach contacts with those at risk. Face-to-face discussions, in particular, were effective in conveying important information, correcting false beliefs and prejudices, and improving the level of knowledge in order to prevent further HIV infections. The distribution of condoms in bars, discos, brothels, saunas, and on the street as well as the distribution of sterile needles in the drug scene were considered by the outreach workers to be very important. (See Gusy *et al.*, 1994.)

Psychosocial support and counselling of HIV-infected drug users   This pilot programme was intended to motivate drug users to make use of counselling services. Specific help was offered to addicts who had developed AIDS and to their families. Twenty-seven staff positions at eighteen drug counselling centres were funded by the programme. Co-operation with the local public health departments and with self-help groups was sought and maintained. (See Schumann *et al.*, 1993.)

AIDS and children   This pilot programme established close links between clinical research, in-patient treatment, out-patient services and psychosocial and nursing care. The goal of this programme was to research the disease and its course, to establish diagnostic methods and therapy approaches, and to observe the epidemiological development of AIDS in children. The programme's key psychosocial objective was developing optimum care for affected families and children. This included identifying and supporting suitable caregivers for the children, should the need arise. Paediatricians, gynaecologists, psychologists, social workers, nurses and nurses aides worked together in this pilot programme. (See Bundesministerium für Gesundheit, 1994.)

Women and AIDS   This pilot programme addressed the special problems of women with respect to AIDS. The areas of emphasis were sexuality, pregnancy, drug addiction, prostitution, and the proper development and establishment of care structures. Medical issues focused on the course of pregnancy in HIV-infected women and the effects of genital infections on the transmission of the virus. In the psychosocial part of the programme, types of support designed specifically for women, including counselling, were identified and their effectiveness investigated. (See Leopold and Steffan, 1994; Schäfer, undated; Friedrich, 1993.)

The pilot programme *Expansion of Outpatient Services for AIDS Patients Within the Framework of Social Service Centres* was a mainstay of the Emergency Programme to Fight AIDS. The programme helped to clarify the specific conditions under which the motto 'as much in-patient care as necessary, as much out-patient care as possible' could be implemented in the management of patients with HIV and AIDS. The experience gained in the programme was an important decision-making tool. State and local governments were prompted to continue this support service, in accordance with the level of demand present in 1992, and to negotiate viable financing regulations with the health insurance companies. (See Schaeffer, Chapter 17, for the results of related research.)

Many elements of the pilot programmes initially evolved from experiences of failure rather than success. Learning from the problems encountered, a further training scheme was created exclusively for all of the approximately 700 professional staff of the pilot projects. Through this process, the latest medical, psychosocial, and nursing know-how regarding AIDS was conveyed as well as information concerning the basic structures of the public health system and the relevant legal and administrative issues. This added training proved to be very helpful for the work in the field. Participation in the course was mandatory and included staff from the various Länder and regions of the country.

Since funding for pilot projects by the Federal Government is time-limited, the Länder eventually had to decide which projects merited further funding so as to ensure the continued implementation of long-term goals and a demand-based provision of services. The statutory health insurance funds were also obliged to share the costs of these endeavours.

Following the unification of the country, the Federal Government immediately initiated a special AIDS prevention programme for the former East Germany. This initiative was devised to help organise effective counselling and support structures there. The Deutsche AIDS-Hilfe invested great effort in implementing outreach-based prevention activities sponsored by the Federal Government. (See Herrn, Chapter 13, for a discussion of prevention in the former East Germany.)

Research

The Federal Government's public health research policy seeks to respond to specific needs of the general population. The focus of its 'Health Research 2000' programme is biomedical research with special attention being paid to aspects of health policy. The federal funding serves health and research policy goals in the context of the constitutional duties incumbent on the Federal Government. In view of the vast field of university-based health research which is under the jurisdiction of the Länder, funding is based on the subsidiarity principle. (See Wright, Chapter 2, concerning the concept of subsidiarity.) The programme is jointly financed by the Federal Ministry for Education and Research (BMBF) and the Federal Ministry for Health (BMG).[2]

In the past, AIDS research was funded by the former Federal Ministry for Research and Technology (BMFT) as an independent research budget item. Since

1994, funds have been appropriated for AIDS research within the framework of the health research programme under the rubric of infectious diseases. Expert consultants are included in decisions regarding the allocation of research funds. Funding has included support for basic research in the social sciences which was incorporated into the programme in 1989. This priority area was to provide knowledge to complement the findings of the evaluative research of the national campaign and the practice-oriented research regarding HIV prevention and care.

In 1987, funding of clinical research started with an ad hoc programme launched by the Federal Ministry for Health. In 1991, this was continued under the title 'The Intensification of Clinical Research' (IdkF). Initially, twenty-seven treatment centres and clinics participated in this programme, these institutions caring for more than half of all AIDS patients in the country. Research projects were planned and implemented as a multi-centre effort comprising the therapeutic management of HIV infection, the evaluation of micro-biological diagnostics, therapy of the attendant opportunistic infections, and the investigation of epidemiological aspects of the disease. Ultimately these projects have substantially contributed to standardising practices for the care and treatment of HIV infected persons and AIDS patients in Germany.

International co-operation in the field of AIDS research is considered to be very important. German working groups and institutions continue to play a major role in the AIDS research programme sponsored by the European Union.

The Federal Ministry for Health primarily funds practice-oriented research, including the collection of epidemiological data and other information which provide a more accurate picture of the course of the disease. In addition, population surveys are commissioned on a regular basis, tracking sexual behaviour and risk exposure in the country as a whole as well as in individual sub-groups. Psychosocial studies are also financed which investigate the consequences of HIV and AIDS for the individual, specific groups, and the population at large as well as the results of strategies being developed to prevent and cope with the disease. (For examples of research commissioned by the Government see Bochow, Chapter 12 and Pott, Chapter 6.)

The research on sexual behaviour has two aspects. The sexual behaviour of the general population of men and women in Germany is being followed with the aim of developing ways to change infection-relevant sexual practices and behavioural patterns through education and counselling. At the same time, the behaviour of homosexuals, the clients of prostitutes, sex tourists and non-monogamous persons, among others, are being studied in a target-group specific manner to discover ways of intervening for these particular populations. The obstacles and the forms of resistance which prevent appropriate communication about AIDS and protection follow-through are being especially examined. These investigations showed, for example, that partners in new relationships or in 'holiday love affairs' often dispense with the use of condoms (Kleiber and Wilke, 1995).

In addition to the above, social science research is conducted on people with HIV/AIDS in an attempt to analyse the development of prejudices and stigmatisation processes in society and the ways in which the general public ostracises those affected. An important focus of this work is examining how these processes can be influenced through educational measures as well as identifying the communication structures, patterns of social exchange, and life-styles that can be important for prevention of this dynamic (Kleiber and Pant, 1996; Gerhards and Schmidt, 1992; Kleiber and Velten, 1994; Dannecker, 1990; see also Jacob *et al.*, Chapter 9).

The Federal Centre for Health Education (BZgA) participates in international research projects that compare knowledge, attitudes and protective behaviour on the European level.

In addition, evaluation studies are being carried out. Evaluation serves to check whether political and practical measures have a positive effect. Changes in attitudes and behaviour are the specific topics of study. A primary goal is to determine whether the number of new infections has declined as a result of the intervention action taken. A large portion of the studies supported by the Federal Ministry for Health have been serving this aim. Evaluation studies have also been conducted in several Länder. Representative surveys, conducted on behalf of the Ministry or the BZgA by Allensbach, Basis Research, FORSA and other polling institutes, as well as targeted comparative surveys are among the primary methods of evaluation.

Finally, the national German AIDS conferences serve to consolidate findings obtained from research and practice. These meetings receive substantial funding from the Federal Government.

Additional measures

The issue of reporting people with HIV/AIDS by name for the purposes of registration has been laid to rest. Experience has shown that the decision to opt for anonymous reporting was correct. What is more, the planned revision of the Federal Law on Communicable Diseases (*Bundesseuchengesetz*) will transform current regulations into a state-of-the-art piece of legislation called the Act on the Protection Against Infectious Diseases. This new law will also not provide for any reporting of infected persons by name. A new feature of the revised law is that not only diagnosed cases but also the identification of pathogens through laboratory tests will be under a mandatory reporting requirement. It will also be necessary to supply more information about the infection, for example, data concerning the probable source of infection. The underlying aim of the new law is to detect and control any risks for infection as they emerge in the population. Information about infection risks and preventive behaviour is important for the protection against epidemics on the national level. Impressive evidence for the effectiveness of such strategies has been furnished by the information campaigns and education efforts in preventing the spread of HIV. (See Pott, Chapter 6.) As a result of these findings, the provision of information and education will be written into the new Act as an obligation of the State. Adequate education implies that competent bodies in the health sector develop targeted and effective prevention strategies and carry out regular monitoring of efficacy and efficiency. In addition, preventing communicable diseases through improved infection epidemiology is a key aim of the new Act.

To investigate the transmission of HIV via blood and blood products, a committee of inquiry of the German Bundestag was organised. At the initiative of the Federal Ministry for Health, the Humanitarian Emergency Assistance Fund was established in 1994 to compensate those injured through blood and blood products; these moneys were superseded in 1995 by a foundation. A total of 250 million marks was made available by the Federal Government, pharmaceutical companies, Länder governments, and the German Red Cross. (See Frankenberg and Hanebeck, Chapter 4.) Fortunately, the current residual risk of virus transmission through blood products is infinitesimal. Established in 1993 by the Federal Ministry for Health, the working group on blood and blood products contributes to improving further the professional and technical practices in blood donation and transfusion services in Germany. The Transfusion Act of 1 July 1998 has legally defined the essential requirements and duties governing blood donation and transfusion practices.

International co-operation

The strategy of the Federal Government is embedded in an international concept which was articulated by the World Health Organisation (for example, in the Ottawa Charter) and by the Conference of Health Ministers which took place in London in 1988. An important outcome of this Conference was the London Declaration on AIDS Prevention which was endorsed by more than 140 countries. The resolutions of the General Assembly of the United Nations and the WHO on combating and controlling AIDS are also supported in full by the German Government. Close co-operation on health policy also exists on the level of the European Union.

Since 1996, a joint HIV/AIDS control programme of the United Nations called UNAIDS has been in existence, replacing the WHO Global Programme on AIDS (GPA) that had been established in 1987. The Federal Ministry of Health shares in the costs of the UNAIDS programme through voluntary contributions. The Federal Ministry for Economic Co-operation and Development (BMZ) supports UNAIDS as the successor to the former GPA. From 1987 to 1997 alone the BMZ made available 22.9 million marks in trust funds. From 1986 to mid-2000 Germany is making available almost 79 million marks alone for the supra-regional project 'AIDS Control in Developing Countries'. Today, more than half of the health projects funded by Germany worldwide include activities on the prevention and treatment of STDs and HIV infections. What is more, the Federal Government continues to participate in WHO campaigns to control AIDS. This includes measures undertaken by the WHO Regional Office for Europe.

Outlook for the future

We have succeeded – albeit through enormous effort, a high financial input, and in the face of frequently massive criticism – in effectively countering HIV/AIDS.

The people of Germany as a whole were largely opposed to ostracising HIV-infected persons and AIDS patients. The success of the Federal Government's comprehensive and timely AIDS control policy – which has been supported by the Länder governments, numerous institutions, associations, and self-help groups – confirms that the approach embarked upon has been the right one.

With its focus on information, counselling and support the strategy for the control of the immunodeficiency disease AIDS is exemplary in German medical history. For no other disease have education, counselling and support structures become so firmly established as has been the case with AIDS. An immense number of the most varied education materials for different target groups has been made available. However, all those involved in the prevention effort must persevere in order to ensure that the coming generations have the necessary knowledge and motivation to engage in protective behaviour. For this purpose, information about AIDS must be conveyed anew, time and again. The habituation to prevention messages, leading to a situation where preventive behaviour is neglected, must be counteracted. It is also important that prevention messages reach their respective target groups.

New groups which have not attracted much notice to date but which are moving increasingly into the focus of epidemiological attention must also become the subject of preventive efforts. This applies particularly to women, whose proportion among those infected is on the increase, and immigrants, who might not be adequately reached by information about HIV and AIDS which is not adapted to their particular cultures. (See Marcus, Chapter 3.)

The climate of solidarity with those affected and their families must be maintained. Also the strengthening of civil rights for minorities must be defended. It remains one of the important tasks of the Federal Government to continue endeavours in order to secure and consolidate these rights.

Notes

1 In 1991 the Federal Ministry for Youth, Family, Affairs, Women and Health (BMJFFG) was divided into two ministries: the Ministry for Health (BMG) and the Ministry for Family Affairs, Senior Citizens, Women and Youth (BMFSFJ).
2 The Federal Ministry for Education and Research (BMBF) was up until 1998 organised under two seperate: the Ministry for Education and Science (BMBW) and the Ministry for Research and Technology (BMFT).

References

Bundesministerium für Forschung und Technologie (BMFT) (1993) Gesundheitsforschung 2000, Programm der Bundesregierung, Bonn: Bundesministerium für Forschung und Technologie.

Bundesministerium für Gesundheit (BMG) (1994) Modellprogramm AIDS und Kinder – medizinische und psychosoziale Aspekte – Schriftenreihe des Bundesministeriums für Gesundheit, Band 34, Baden-Baden: Nomos Verlagsgesellschaft.

—— (1997) Gesundheit in Deutschland, Bonn: Bundesministerium für Gesundheit.

—— (1999) AIDS-Bekämpfung in Deutschland. Bonn: Bundesministerium für Gesundheit.

Bundesministerium für wirtschaftliche Zusammenarbeit und Entwicklung (BMZ) (1998) HIV/AIDS-Bekämpfung. Eine Antwort auf die Ausbreitung in den Entwicklungs-ländern in BMZ aktuell, Nr. 094/September.

Dannecker, M. (1990) *Homosexuelle Männer und AIDS, Schriftenreihe des Bundesministeriums für Jugend, Familie, Frauen und Gesundheit*, Band 252, Stuttgart, Berlin and Cologne: Verlag W. Kohlhammer.

Deutscher Bundestag (1990) *Abschlußbericht der Enquete-Kommission des Deutschen Bundestages 'Gefahren von AIDS und wirksame Wege zu ihrer Eindämmung, AIDS: Fakten und Konsequenzen'* Zur Sache 90/13. Bonn: Deutscher Bundestag.

Filsinger, D., Schäfer, J. Vollendorf, M. *et al.* (1993) *Supervision in der AIDS-Arbeit.* Freie Universität Berlin, Fachbereich Philosophie und Sozialwissenschaften I, Psychologisches Institut, Berlin: Freie Universität.

Friedrich, M. (1993) *Mädchen und AIDS. Schriftenreihe des Bundesministeriums für Gesundheit*, Band 22, Baden-Baden: Nomos Verlagsgesellschaft.

Gerhards, J. and Schmidt, B. (1992) *Intime Kommunikation. Schriftenreihe des Bundesministeriums für Gesundheit*, Band 11, Baden-Baden: Nomos Verlags-gesellschaft.

Gusy, B., Krauß, G., Schrott, G. and Heckmann, W. (1994) *Aufsuchende Sozialarbeit in der AIDS-Prävention – das Streetworker-Modell, Schriftenreihe des Bundesministeriums für Gesundheit*, Band 21, Baden-Baden: Nomos Verlagsgesellschaft.

Kleiber, D. and Pant, A. (1996) *HIV – Needle-Sharing – Sex. Schriftenreihe des Bundesministeriums für Gesundheit*, Band 69a, Baden-Baden: Nomos Verlags-Gesellschaft.

Kleiber, D. and Velten, D. (1994) *Prostitutionskunden. Schriftenreihe des Bundesmin-isteriums für Gesundheit*, Band 30, Baden-Baden: Nomos Verlagsgesellschaft.

Kleiber, D. and Wilke, M. (1995) AIDS, *Sex und Tourismus. Schriftenreihe des Bundes-ministeriums für Gesundheit*, Band 33, Baden-Baden: Nomos Verlagsgesellschaft.

Leopold, B. and Steffan, E. (1994) *Frauen und AIDS*, Berlin: Sozialpädagogisches Institut.

Schäfer, A. P. A. (undated) *Multizentrische Studie 'Frauen und AIDS'* Berlin: Universitäts-frauenklinik der medizinischen Fakultät der Humboldt Universität.

Schumann, J., Fahrner, E. M. and Niemeck, U. (1993) *Modellprogramm Drogen und AIDS, Schriftenreihe des Bundesministeriums für Gesundheit*, Band 19, Baden-Baden: Nomos Verlagsgesellschaft.

Thoben, I., Müller, D., Angerstein, E. *et al.* (1991) *Großmodell Gesundheitsämter – AIDS. Schriftenreihe des Instituts für Gesundheits-System-Forschung*, Band 38, Kiel: Institut für Gesundheits-System-Forschung.

6 AIDS prevention campaigns for the general public

The work of the Federal Centre for Health Education

Elisabeth Pott

Introduction

Before AIDS, the approach to epidemics of infectious diseases in Germany was regulated by the Federal Law on Communicable Diseases (*Bundesseuchengesetz*) which provides for control and containment strategies, including the compulsory registration of infected persons and, if necessary, compulsory treatment and quarantine. With the appearance of AIDS new strategies were implemented to combat the spread of a contagious disease. The decision not to employ traditional strategies, but to initiate nationwide prevention campaigns based on Social Learning Theory (Bandura, 1986) was a significant step. The decisive factors were the lack of effective treatment options for HIV and the realisation that identifying and isolating people who were infected would be useless because of the long period of latency and the pandemic spread of the disease. Another important issue was that people affected by HIV organised themselves into self-help initiatives. In this way, they gained political influence on the development of a prevention approach which focused on the human needs of the groups most affected, as opposed to the characteristics of the pathogenic agent itself. (See Frankenberg and Hanebeck, Chapter 4; Schilling, Chapter 8.)

It took time for the conflict about AIDS prevention in Germany to coalesce into a consensus position supporting a long-term national AIDS strategy organised as a social learning process, based on the principles of co-operation between the relevant institutions and organisations in the country. (See Frankenberg and Hanebeck, Chapter 4.) AIDS has been and will continue to be a major challenge within the overall modern public health strategy.

The National AIDS Campaign key principles

The main principles of the National AIDS Campaign are:

*   Setting up and maintaining a new public health infrastructure for information, counselling, and care.
*   Co-operation between governmental institutions and non-governmental organisations within the health care sector.

- Division of labour between the various players.
- Action on the federal, state and local levels.
- Acceptance of various lifestyles and the promotion of individual responsibility.
- Exclusion of panic-inducing strategies.
- Evaluation to guide the development of the national campaign.

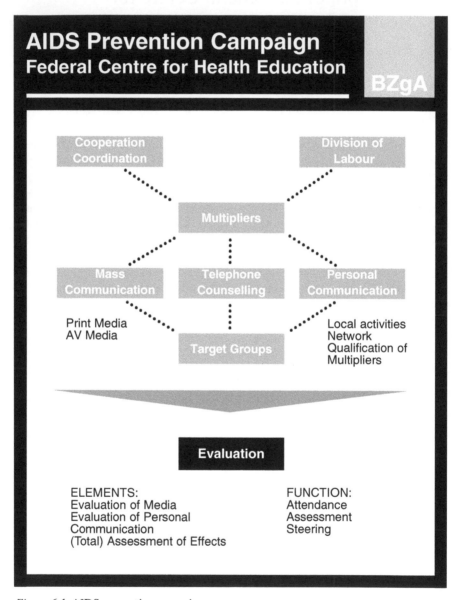

Figure 6.1 AIDS prevention campaign

Note: "Multipliers" refers to those persons who are in a position to pass information on to specific
target groups (for example, professionals with contact with young people, gay men, etc.)

Campaign goals and objectives

Fortunately, a social consensus has been finally achieved on the goals and messages of the AIDS prevention campaign. The entire campaign is intended to curb the further spread of HIV and AIDS as effectively as possible and to contribute to the integration of people with HIV and AIDS into society. This necessitates the following goals:

- Attaining a high level of information in the population about risks for infection.
- Dispelling fears based on incorrect information.
- Motivating people to protect themselves against infection when in risk situations.
- Creating a social climate which opposes the stigmatisation and isolation of people with HIV and AIDS.

In order to meet these goals, the most important objectives of AIDS prevention are:

- Informing about the means of transmission, effective protective measures, the syndrome of AIDS, the course of the disease, the epidemiology of the virus and about HIV testing.
- Motivating protective behaviour which includes discussing barriers to protection, developing communication skills for difficult situations, strengthening personal identity, supporting the ability for self-assertion and promoting responsibility for oneself and for others.
- Promoting solidarity for people with HIV/AIDS; for example, by exposing prejudices and stigmatisation in society and by providing information on the harmlessness of casual social contacts with those infected.

Target groups for AIDS prevention

The AIDS prevention campaign addresses the general population as a whole as well as special target groups, including the primarily affected groups (men who have sex with men and intravenous drug users) as well as women, youth, young adults, the clients of prostitutes, long-distance travellers, and various professional groups who provide prevention and education to diverse segments of the population (for example, nurses, teachers, day-care workers and drug counsellors), here referred to as 'multipliers'.

The prevention needs of the various target groups need to be addressed via specific communication channels. As governmental and other public institutions have only limited access to homosexuals and intravenous drug users, the so-called primarily affected groups in Germany, non-governmental organisations are provided with the resources to design appropriate messages and strategies. Most important is the Deutsche AIDS-Hilfe (DAH), the National German AIDS Organisation, which has established a credibility within these groups by employing insider knowledge of the various lifestyles and by using appropriate language and media. (See Schilling, Chapter 8; Etgeton, Chapter 7.) Acceptance of prevention messages within the general population is, on the other hand, heightened when campaigns are sponsored by a neutral authority such as the Federal Centre for Health Education (BZgA). One finds, therefore, a division of labour on the national level in Germany regarding HIV prevention, with the DAH focusing on the most affected groups and the BZgA designing and implementing strategies for the general population.

Messages

The main slogan of the National Campaign is 'Don't give AIDS a Chance' (*Gib AIDS keine Chance*). The campaign integrates the following messages:

- AIDS is a serious disease without a cure.
- It is largely up to you whether you become infected with HIV, as the main transmission routes are unprotected sexual intercourse and intravenous drug use.
- Therefore, inform yourself, protect yourself and your partner (by using condoms in sexual risk situations), and do not isolate people with HIV and AIDS.

Co-operation

Developing partnerships for co-operation at the national level has been most important for the success of the AIDS prevention campaign. Therefore the Federal Centre for Health Education, a governmental organisation at the national level, decided very early to co-operate with the leading national non-governmental organisation, the Deutsche AIDS-Hilfe, delegating certain aspects of the AIDS prevention campaign to this partner. The idea behind this co-operation was that a self-help organisation of people primarily affected with AIDS (especially homosexual and bisexual men) would have more credibility and therefore find more acceptance in these communities. Because of its high standing in the eyes of the general public, the Federal Centre for Health Education, as a government authority, focused its work on the needs of the (predominantly heterosexual) general public.

With the co-operation between the BZgA and the DAH as a foundation, an entire network of collaboration was established with other partners. In the federalist political system of Germany, the individual states have played a most significant role in these ongoing relationships. Other important partners have included: local public health authorities, other federal ministries, the World Health Organisation, UNAIDS, the European Union, scientific institutes (most notably the AIDS Centre at the Robert Koch Institute in Berlin) and other national associations.

Our experience has shown that successful education campaigns on the population level are possible when:

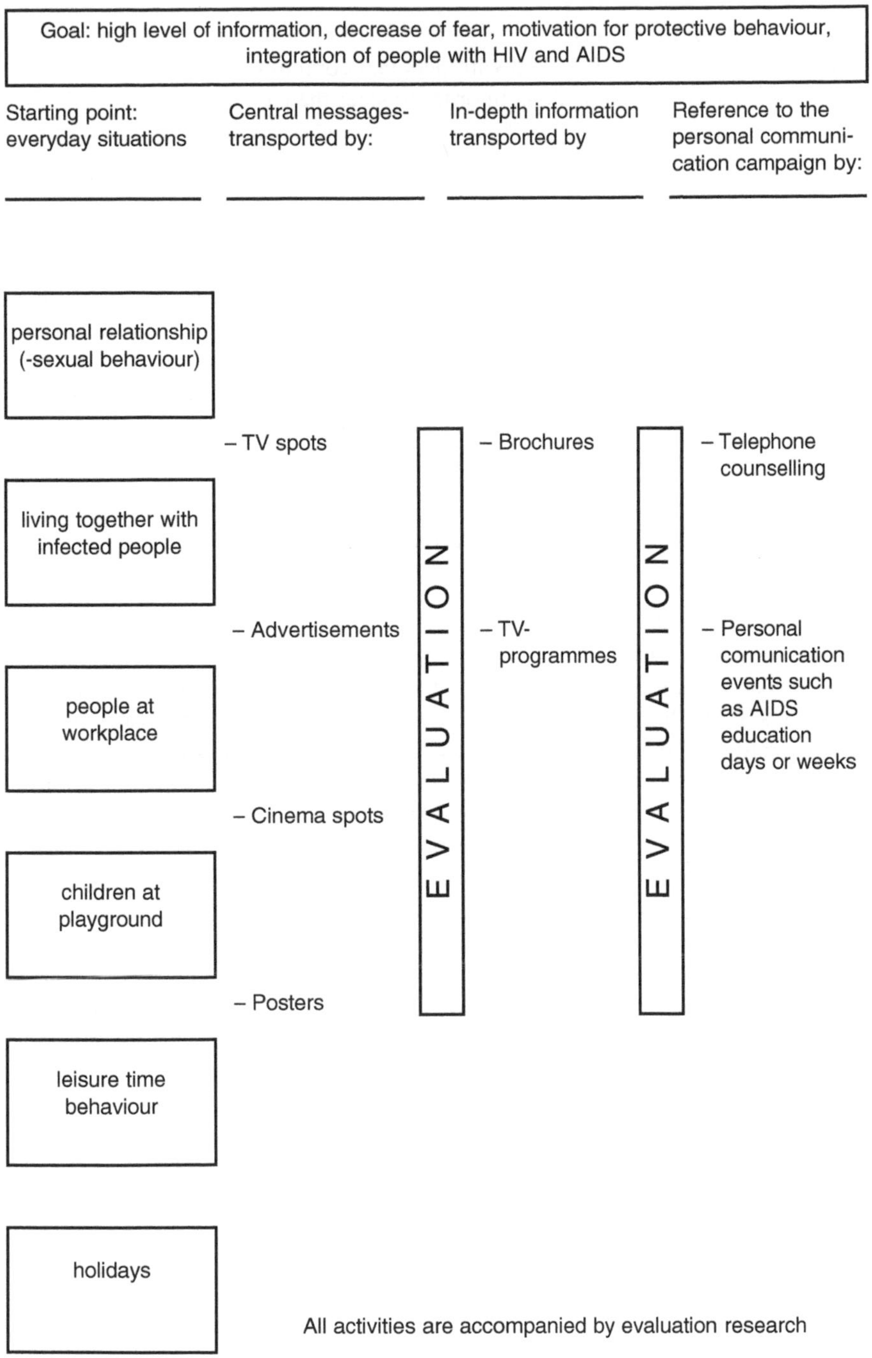

Goal: high level of information, decrease of fear, motivation for protective behaviour, integration of people with HIV and AIDS			
Starting point: everyday situations	Central messages-transported by:	In-depth information transported by	Reference to the personal communication campaign by:

personal relationship (-sexual behaviour)

living together with infected people

people at workplace

children at playground

leisure time behaviour

holidays

– TV spots

– Advertisements

– Cinema spots

– Posters

E V A L U A T I O N

– Brochures

– TV-programmes

E V A L U A T I O N

– Telephone counselling

– Personal comunication events such as AIDS education days or weeks

All activities are accompanied by evaluation research

Figure 6.2 Mass media campaign

- A campaign is preceded by careful problem analysis of the audience and the message.
- Target groups are defined.
- Mass communication is linked with personal communication.
- Continuous evaluation is done in order to steer the campaign.

Capacity building

Within a modern health education campaign a social learning process has to be established which will remain effective in the long term. The aim of the National AIDS Campaign in Germany was to strengthen individuals' skills, thus strengthening their ability to act and to assert their personal responsibility. To achieve this goal, the infrastructure for a new kind of public health strategy had to be developed. The result was a complex information and education approach consisting of several elements of mass communication, interpersonal communication and one-to-one counselling.

Personal communication: more self-determination regarding one's health

An innovative element has been the personal communication component of the national campaign. The concept of personal communication was developed in order to close the gap between the mass media and the one-to-one counselling components. It had become evident that people could only relate messages in the mass media to their individual situation by means of personal conversations with others in their social environment. We sought to promote such conversations through this component of the campaign. Although it was important for people to talk about AIDS as a disease, it was even more relevant for discussions to take place regarding problem areas such as: sexuality, partnership, responsibility, love and solidarity with infected and ill people. Through such conversations taboo subjects could be addressed, thereby reducing barriers to protective behaviour.

This component of the campaign requires promoting discussions which are frank but at the same time sensitive to the life style and language of the different target groups. Only by openly presenting the issues at hand is it possible to motivate and educate people on how to form their own opinions, how to assess their situation realistically, and how to make responsible decisions for themselves. The aim of modern health promotion and education strategies must be enabling people to gain more control of their own health. This was the approach of the interpersonal communication campaign: Not to give advice or ready-made answers for good health, but to create a basis for responsible decisions and dialogue. Within the campaign we address specific risk situations which individuals can relate to their own lives, thus enabling them to recognise the dangers in advance and to react to concrete situations in a realistic way, appropriate to their particular lifestyles. Individual are thus enabled to gain control of the problem of AIDS in their own lives and to develop their own personalised options for action. The development of a personal prevention strategy is necessary in order to address feelings of helplessness and powerlessness, and to correct decisions based on false information.

A good example for this kind of practical work with young people is the so-called 'Hands-On Course'. The BZgA offers this course to its co-operative partners in the form of a project week in which approximately 500 participants can be reached. Prevention counsellors, acting on behalf of the BZgA, support the co-operative partners in preparing and implementing the project. This project is especially suitable for students between the ages of 12 and 16, young people no longer in school, trainers in companies and soldiers in basic training.

There are six play stations, each station dealing with certain aspects of AIDS in the form of self-contained discussion units. The participants can take part in facilitated discussions, focusing particularly on their personal protective behaviour for HIV and on questions of responsibility and solidarity towards people with HIV/AIDS (for example, colleagues in the workplace). The topics of the six play stations are:

- Love, sexuality, and protection against HIV.
- Protection against unwanted pregnancy, STD's, and HIV.
- Using condoms.
- Body language and sexuality.
- Living with HIV/AIDS in the workplace.
- Information station.

Telephone counselling

An anonymous telephone hotline on AIDS was set up at the Federal Centre for Health Education in 1987. The telephone number was first publicised through ten television spots which launched the national campaign in May of the same year. Later on the hotline number was publicised through advertisements, posters, further television and cinema spots, and using all the other common mass media materials. A low-threshold service was thus established which enabled the BZgA to deal directly and individually with the questions, worries and fears of the population. The telephone hotline – which operates seven days a week and thus also fills the counselling gap on weekends – enables individuals to relate the information provided in the mass media to their individual situation and to their personal problems, thus helping callers to translate prevention information into concrete action. There continues to be a strong response to this service.

Promoting joint actions

AIDS Information Days are an example of the kind of events which bring together interested members of the public and various prevention partners for dialogue and discussion on the local level. In close co-operation with local community-based organisations, the information and education events are planned, implemented and

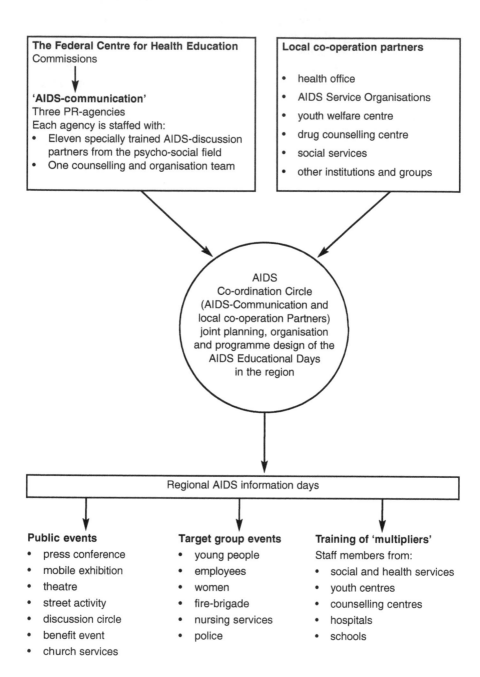

The Federal Centre for Health Education
Commissions

↓

'AIDS-communication'
Three PR-agencies
Each agency is staffed with:
- Eleven specially trained AIDS-discussion partners from the psycho-social field
- One counselling and organisation team

Local co-operation partners

- health office
- AIDS Service Organisations
- youth welfare centre
- drug counselling centre
- social services
- other institutions and groups

AIDS
Co-ordination Circle
(AIDS-Communication and local co-operation Partners)
joint planning, organisation and programme design of the AIDS Educational Days in the region

Regional AIDS information days

Public events
- press conference
- mobile exhibition
- theatre
- street activity
- discussion circle
- benefit event
- church services

Target group events
- young people
- employees
- women
- fire-brigade
- nursing services
- police

Training of 'multipliers'
Staff members from:
- social and health services
- youth centres
- counselling centres
- hospitals
- schools

Figure 6.3 Personal communication campaign

evaluated by the BZgA. These events include a variety of activities, such as booths on the street, concerts, disco nights, theatre performances, and round table discussions focused on the subject of AIDS. The range of interaction includes everything from discussions in larger groups to confidential chats. Through such joint projects we are able to meet the goal of strengthening co-operation while actively promoting community-oriented approaches.

As a result of joint project planning and implementation, innovations in public health have been achieved. Most importantly, co-operation between the governmental and the non-governmental sectors has assumed a new level of importance which did not exist in Germany prior to the development of the National AIDS Campaign. In addition, public health authorities have taken on a more active role in providing prevention information to the public, going beyond their traditional containment and control functions in response to STDs. This has had a large impact on improving the image of the local public health authorities in the eyes of the general population.

Solidarity

Involving public figures in certain aspects of AIDS education – such as artists and politicians – can lead to increased solidarity and support for people with HIV/AIDS. The National Campaign has been built on the premise that social integration, self-confidence, and self-esteem are important preconditions for protective behaviour. For this reason, promoting and supporting solidarity with HIV-positive people and AIDS patients was an important component from the beginning. The discussion has not been limited to the illness itself. In response to suggestions from members of the target groups and other co-operative partners, a wide range of subjects such as ethics, social norms and values, and the personal dimension of the disease have been discussed.

Evaluation

Since 1987 the BZgA has financed ongoing research of the various aspects of the National AIDS Campaign. The following elements of the campaign have been subject to evaluation: specific media components, telephone counselling, the interpersonal communication component and the combined effects of all activities of the National Campaign as a whole. An important element in the evaluative process has been annual surveys on representative national samples to monitor population changes in knowledge, attitudes and behaviour regarding AIDS (for example, BZgA 1988, 1998).

We have sought to measure the success of the campaign by monitoring certain parameters in the population over time:

- Level of knowledge about infection risks.
- Change in social attitudes toward people with HIV and AIDS.
- Protective behaviour for HIV, especially the use of condoms during sexual contact with new partners whose infection status is unknown.

- Condom purchase.
- Incidence of STDs (other than HIV).
- Incidence of HIV.
- Condom use in general.

The results of the last evaluation, conducted in 1998, reveal the following (BZgA, 1998):

- Over 90 per cent of the population knows how HIV is transmitted and how they can protect themselves against infection.
- The social acceptance and solidarity for people with HIV/AIDS has improved. In 1985, before the education campaign was set up, more than one third (36 per cent) of the population more than 16 years old were of the opinion that AIDS patients should not have contact to anyone except medical personnel and relatives. In 1998 only a relatively small portion of the population expressed ostracising and discriminating opinions (approximately 4 per cent).
- The intention for protective behaviour is high (intention viewed here as a prerequisite for behaviour).
- Protective behaviour has increased steadily over the course of the campaign, especially in those groups who are most at risk. In 1998, 72 per cent of single men and women aged 45 years or younger used condoms (in 1988: 58 per cent). In 1998, 76 per cent of people with several sexual partners (in 1988: 54 per cent) and 84 per cent of young people between 16 and 20 years used condoms (in 1988: 59 per cent).

Condom purchase

The trend in condom purchase corresponds to that found in protective behaviour. In the 1984 survey, 84 million condoms were sold; in 1998 the figure rose to 200 million.

Incidence of STDs

The number of reported STD cases as documented by the Federal Office of Statistics shows a clear decreasing trend since 1985 (Statistisches Bundesamt, 1997; Marcus, Chapter 3). For example, there were 6.5 cases of syphilis in 1985 for every 100,000 inhabitants; this dropped to 1.4 per 100,000 in 1997. In the case of gonorrhoea we notice an even greater decrease with 60.2/100,000 cases reported in 1985 and 3.6/100,000 in 1997.

Incidence of HIV

The AIDS surveillance program of the Robert Koch Institute in Berlin reports a stable epidemiological pattern, with an incidence of approximately 2,000–2,500 per year. (See Marcus, Chapter 3.)

Condom use: the first signs of a reverse trend

Since 1996 we have, however, noticed a stagnation in the trend toward increased condom use. In fact, results since 1998 show a reverse trend developing, with less protective behaviour among persons with several partners. This development parallels a trend since 1994 in information and communication behaviour.

That means that the declining dissemination of AIDS prevention media obviously has an impact on the communication behaviour of the population. For example, the interpersonal communication on the subject of AIDS among friends and acquaintances is declining. As a consequence, protective behaviour is no longer increasing; there is a stagnation and partly a decrease in behaviour noticed in the last years. Among occasional condom users there is a very great number of people (34 per cent) who are no longer reached by the media of the AIDS campaign.

We believe this is due to severe funding cuts from the Federal Government in recent years which have limited our ability to reach many segments of the population, particularly groups with a high risk for infection. There is also less media attention focused on AIDS, in general. As a result, AIDS is a less important topic in people's private lives, leading to a decline in protective behaviour. Therefore, we regretfully cannot report further progress in the effects of the National Campaign in recent years.

Although there is still a relatively high level of protective behaviour in Germany in the general population, we have to consider the trends in recent years to be a clear warning not to lessen efforts in the field of prevention.

Conclusion

The initial forecasts concerning the dramatic spread of HIV in the German population have been successfully averted due to several factors, including the National AIDS Campaign. The epidemiological situation has shown such a stable course in recent years that there has been increasing discussion concerning the normalisation of AIDS. (See Rosenbrock *et al.*, Chapter 20.) From our perspective, normalisation means that society has become aware of AIDS and that most people are familiar with how to prevent its transmission. The discussion about normalisation is an important consequence of the progress made in medical research regarding the treatment of HIV/AIDS, although neither a vaccine nor a cure has been found. HIV/AIDS is slowly becoming a chronic disease with which one can live for several years: albeit with serious symptoms for several people affected. This tendency toward normalisation means also that there is a danger of underestimating the necessity for maintaining the level prevention work which has succeeded over the years. Those in charge of deciding future funding need to look carefully at what resources are necessary to maintain the AIDS prevention infrastructure so as to sustain the relatively good epidemiological situation in Germany. In addition, the experience gained in developing the innovative and successful public health policy in the field of AIDS should be used as a model for other fields of health and social problems.

References

Bandura, A. (1986) *Social Foundations of Thought and Action: Social Cognitive Theory*, Englewood Cliffs, N.Y.: Prentice Hall.

Bundeszentrale für gesundheitliche Aufklärung (BZgA) (1996) 'Aspekte der bundesweiten AIDS-Präventionskampagne', Internationalen AIDS-Konferenz in Vancouver, 07. – 12. Juli 1996, Cologne: BZgA.

—— (1988) Wiederholungsbefragung 'AIDS im öffentlichen Bewußtsein der Bundesrepublik 1988', Cologne: BZgA.

—— (1998) Wiederholungsbefragung 'AIDS im öffentlichen Bewußtsein der Bundesrepublik 1998', Cologne: BZgA.

Deutscher Bundestag (1990) 'AIDS: Fakten und Konsequenzen', Endbericht der Enquete-Kommission des 11. Deutschen Bundestages 'Gefahren von AIDS und wirksame Wege zu ihrer Eindämmung', Bonn: Deutscher Bundestag.

Rosenbrock, R. (1987) *AIDS kann schneller besiegt werden. Gesundheitspolitik am Beispiel einer Infektionskrankheit*, Hamburg: VSA-Verlag.

—— (1992) 'AIDS: Fragen und Lehren für Public Health. WZB-Forschung', discussion paper, Berlin: Wissenschaftszentrum Berlin (WZB).

Statistisches Bundesamt (1997) *Fachserie 12, Reihe 2, Meldepflichtige Krankheiten*, Wiesbaden: Statistisches Bundesamt.

7 Structural prevention

The basis for a critical approach to health promotion

Stefan Etgeton

In the beginning

The first step in the debate defining the politically and strategically appropriate way to go about providing HIV and AIDS prevention in Germany came to a close in 1987. The decision was made to forego the traditional and repressive control and containment measures typically implemented in response to infectious diseases in favour of health learning strategies according to the principles of health promotion. This decision was made relatively early in Germany. (See Frankenberg and Hanebeck, Chapter 4; Schilling, Chapter 8.) But this was only the first step.

As soon as it was decided to go the way of informational and motivational strategies to fight the epidemic, the debate began concerning the appropriate learning strategy to adopt. At the time there were two schools of thought. The behaviourists wanted to condition people through information campaigns and training programs with the goal of consistent patterns of behaviour being adopted so as to prevent as many new infections as possible. On the other side of the debate were the depth psychologists who, in deference to the often tricky strategies employed by unconscious desires, discussed the price to be paid for changing sexual practices, namely sensual deprivation and the fetters of conformity. They warned that an inevitable unconscious resistance needs to be taken into account by any prevention strategy.

In applying the tenets of Critical Theory to sexual science we can surmise that any information campaign lacking an emancipatory character runs the danger of disempowering people to act for themselves. Anyone who wants to create lasting behaviour change and thereby assist the person in internalising these changes must be prepared to affect the situation and the environment in which the behaviour takes place. The mechanical conditioning of response patterns through behaviourist approaches only affects the superficial level of the behaviour and necessarily results in misguided strategies or in repressive measures. In general, the local AIDS Service Organisations (ASOs), the AIDS-Hilfen, have incorporated into their work perspectives from both behaviourism and depth psychology. The 'pure teaching' of the Deutsche AIDS-Hilfe, the National German AIDS Organisation, has, however, been clearly based on the latter.

The ability to manage one's own risks properly depends upon more than just behaviour. The structures in which people live – society, culture and family – are as important as their knowledge and attitudes regarding what they actually do. Therefore prevention strategies seek to improve the social, political, and cultural contexts in which people live and love so as to enable the individual to better managing his/her own specific risks. The word 'structure' seemed appropriate in the 1980s to describe these dimensions. It was very common then to talk about structural causes, for example, 'structural violence', which was seen as the cause of violent behaviour and thus the appropriate focus for violence prevention. It was a short step to transfer this thinking to health promotion when coining the phrase *structural prevention*.

From this discussion crystallised the first principle of structural prevention, namely: the unity of prevention at the individual behavioural level and at the level of the social environmental (in German: *Verhaltens- und Verhältnisprävention*). However, defining this principle raised a host of new problems, as discussed in this chapter.

Emancipation is prevention

The phrase emancipation is prevention soon became a leitmotif for structural prevention. What is meant by this phrase is that emancipation is a requirement for the long-term success of prevention. Even though hindering HIV infection was the primary goal of the work, it was important to identify the social conditions necessary for prevention to succeed. This position reflects the principle of Critical Theory that the improvement of individual segments of society is only possible through changing society as a whole, or in the words of Adorno (1951) 'There is no emancipation without the emancipation of society'. What this means concretely for prevention is that, using gay men as an example, health promotion is only possible through promoting self-awareness, removing marginalisation and discrimination, and preserving and valuing the subculture – most importantly, those aspects of the subculture generally viewed by society as dirty or undesirable. It is only through subcultural venues and organisations that the majority of gay men can be reached. Protecting these places as havens for gay men is therefore a requirement for the success of prevention messages placed there.

Such an abstract discussion of an all-encompassing emancipation of society as being the prerequisite for prevention can quickly result in frustration and overestimating what is possible. To be consistent, one could argue that we need to forgo prevention activities altogether until society has been completely emancipated. The thesis 'emancipation is prevention' articulates an ambitious and ingenious standard, which can only be maintained as long as the logic of prevention and emancipation are allowed to meld and all inconsistencies are ignored. In real life, however, this standard can lead to exaggerated expectations, excessive demands on oneself, and to a cynical, hypocritical stance. Even in the absence of the progress made regarding the emancipation of gay men and drug users, the ASOs in Germany, of course, would have continued to do prevention work, doing the right thing in the wrong context. (See Rosenbrock, Chapter 19; Schilling, Chapter 8; Barsch, Chapter 14; Frankenberg and Hanebeck, Chapter 4.) Currently we observe an epidemiological shift among gay men to an increased burden on marginalised men; that is, the less attractive, the less educated, the less wealthy, the less socially and culturally integrated are more at risk than the emancipated, middle-class, 'normal' gay man. (See Bochow, Chapter 12.) The problem with the concept of a preventive emancipation is that it is most commonly oriented to the self-aware, middle-class gay man, thus blinding us to the demands of the emerging epidemics among other (gay) populations.

One could try turning the equation around to read 'prevention is emancipation'. Indeed a critical theory of health would reject this idea because a preventive act which is essentially a reaction to epidemiological necessity would seldom have an emancipatory effect. However, when one considers the history of the German ASO movement and its consequences, it can hardly be disputed that HIV prevention has had numerous emancipatory results. The 'solidarity of the marginalised' paid off. When one argues that emancipation is a requirement for a long-lasting prevention success, then this sets the stage for progress in terms of emancipation when doing prevention work. Because of the AIDS issue an infrastructure has come into being (for example, gay information and contact centres) and certain other developments have taken place (for example, methadone maintenance) which would not have happened, or at least would not have happened so quickly, if it were not for AIDS and the ASOs. At the same time there is the risk that the instrumentalisation of health promotion in order to achieve political emancipation can lead to emancipation being equated with health. This can result in emancipatory structures being reduced to vehicles for disease prevention. Prevention is not *per se* a means toward emancipation, although it can at times serve that purpose.

When the public authorities at both the state and national level begin to examine more closely the activities of the ASOs in light of their mandate, it is precisely the emancipatory effects of HIV prevention which are called increasingly into question as being outside of the original intent of the funding. Although this external pressure is being primarily dictated by shortfalls in government budgets, it presents the opportunity for the ASOs to articulate more precisely the tasks and services which they provide and thereby to create their own definition of quality in prevention work. This process may also be an opportunity for the ASOs to value their professionalism as a form of political success, as opposed to their general tendency of seeing their work as being insufficient in light of the high ideal of emancipation.

The methods of emancipatory work and of health promotion are not necessarily compatible. Only when the inherent differences between prevention and emancipation are made clear, as in our examination of the phrase 'emancipation is prevention', is it possible to identify the blindness of prevention, the illusion of emancipation, and the repressive potential in mixing emancipation and health together. It is helpful to qualify the relationship between the two by stating that emancipation is a methodological criterion for health promotion *ex negativo*. No prevention measure – be it successful or not – which reduces the competence and self-determination of individuals or groups to disease prevention meets this criterion. This formulation implies a recognition of the boundaries of AIDS work. If the emancipation of society as a whole is neither an absolute requirement for, nor a necessary effect of prevention, then the primary task of the ASOs is solely health promotion in the most comprehensive sense, but it is a health promotion characterised by an integration of the emancipation principle.

AIDS work takes place where desire, pleasure, and health meet – or fail to meet. It is political to the extent that these issues are controversial in society. The emancipatory character of prevention has to do with the philosophical and practical manner with which these controversies are handled. Essentially, this is dependent on the utopian ideal of a society free to explore its sensuality, a perspective which has more to do with political intervention than with the behaviour of specific individuals. To put it another way: the focus of AIDS work is not emancipating society, a goal which is well beyond the movement's capability; however, the ASOs can intervene in such a way as to promote rather than hinder all developments in the service of emancipation. What concrete forms this activity should take needs to be considered within the specific situation.

The criterion of health promotion in the service of emancipation means in a pro-active sense: activating, supporting and maintaining, to the fullest extent possible, people's self-healing and self-help potential, and promoting their ability to enjoy all the pleasures possible in the meantime. In the reactive sense, the criterion means: opposing all preventive measures which disregard the wealth of desire or lead to the marginalisation, disempowerment, degradation, or injury of people affected by HIV/AIDS, living or deceased. Observing this criterion is not only a professional requirement for long-lasting success in health promotion, but also entails an ethical dimension for the ASOs as advocates for people with HIV/AIDS. This ethical dimension is crucial if the increasing professionalism of the ASOs is to reflect their original mission.

A system of mutual respect

The emancipatory principle described by the unity of prevention at the individual behavioural level and at the level of the social environment had additional implications for the development of the concept of structural prevention. The identity of ASOs as self-help organisations for people with HIV/AIDS led to a modification in how the primary prevention of HIV was conceptualised. At the national level, within the Deutsche AIDS-Hilfe itself, this was realised in the form of a power shift; ensuring the representation of people with HIV on the board of directors was meant to reflect who had a say within the organisation. This resulted in all primary prevention measures needing to justify themselves to HIV positive board members, a group of people for whom they were not originally designed. In effect, this process turned out to be a way to ensure that new infections would not be combated at any price, for example, by blaming the 'victim'.

The losses and injuries suffered by people already living with HIV/AIDS would not be overlooked in the zeal to achieve success in primary prevention. This apparent contradiction – valuing the experiences of those infected while seeking to prevent the spread of the disease – has not compromised the primary prevention efforts of the ASOs; in fact, this dual position has increased the credibility of prevention efforts, both within and outside the organisations.

The argument that people living with the disease need to bear with the unavoidable discomfort of the messages promoted in prevention campaigns has not met with much resonance in German ASOs. Avoiding the use of dramatic depictions of illness and death has also shown itself to be state of the art, as fear is not the proper vehicle for promoting lasting health. In recent years other health campaigns, for example those against smoking, have also taken leave from using the 'God is with us' approach. Even in light of the new therapies for HIV and the general perception that AIDS is no longer a major problem in Germany, there is no reason to deviate from the path of mutual respect between the infected and the non-infected which has led to success.

This policy of mutual respect has thus led to a unity of primary, secondary and tertiary prevention which has had consequences for the practical services provided by the ASOs. As a whole, the movement addresses everything from prevention to hospice services, although each individual ASO may not have the capacity to cover all the various areas.

Structural prevention has shown itself to be a flexible concept with both inductive and deductive components. Inductively, the concept finds expression in the principles for the work of the ASOs, based on their concrete experience with prevention at all three levels as well as with the individual and societal factors affecting preventive behaviour. Structural prevention is the 'orthodox teaching' of the ASOs which brings together the political, the professional and the experiential (living with the disease). Deductively, the input from critical perspectives in the health sciences places the work of the ASOs within the context of modern public health theory in the spirit of the WHO Ottawa Charter (WHO, 1986). The AIDS service movement in Germany has essentially been a pilot project for the 'New Deal' in public health in that the principles of health promotion were realised within community-based practice. The term health promotion is a more comprehensive term than prevention, the latter still encumbered by the negative logic of protection, deterrence, and avoidance. Health promotion is inherently positive; that is, it supports a consistent and personally acceptable strategy of physical, psychological, and social well-being. However, the concept of health as defined by the WHO (1986) is far too broad, compromising the ability of health promotion to identify a realistic focus for activity.

Health promotion and self-help as one

In the development of the theoretical foundation for the work of the ASOs which we have been describing thus far, there is a third important theme which deals with the very heart of the AIDS service movement. This is the relationship between professionalism and the role of people with HIV/AIDS, in other words the relationship between health promotion and self-help. In the work of the ASOs conflicts often arise between the staff and those who feel themselves being forced into the client role. 'Help yourself, otherwise you'll be at the mercy of your social worker' is a joke making its way around the ASOs, illustrating the conflict between 'professional' health promotion and the alternative of self-help. A critical perspective within health promotion uses an emancipatory focus to join prevention and self-help at the conceptual and professional levels.

The original idea of AIDS-Hilfe combined both elements in that gay men attempted to provide information to other gay men about the new political and health crisis while working together to achieve a united response. (see Schilling, Chapter 8.) From the beginning the ASO movement in Germany felt itself obliged to work in the service of a larger collective body: gay men, drug users, at-risk women and people with HIV/AIDS. Although it has been complicated to determine the concrete interests of these groups, the attempt to do so has had a regulatory function for the work of the ASOs. More recently, there is a growing critique that the AIDS service movement in Germany is no longer self-help oriented in the true sense of the word. At the same time the status of self-help within ASOs is still an important issue; that is, whether self-help is an essential professional standard, an optional service, or a non-existent entity. With emancipation as the basis for the work, health promotion and personal initiative belong together, both in theory and practice. Although prevention at all three levels and at both the individual and social levels can be implemented 'from above', the approach of an emancipatory health promotion needs to activate, strengthen, and maintain the potential for self-help and self-healing 'from below' to the full extent possible.

Also important is the way in which the AIDS service movement defines itself and the groups to which it has an obligation. In the beginning of the movement, primary prevention was the focus at a time when the number of HIV-positive people was still relatively small. Historically gay men, most of whom were untested or HIV-negative, founded the movement; however, the very heterogeneous group of people with HIV/AIDS has over time taken centre stage. Whereas in the beginning of AIDS work the emphasis was on human rights, equality and anti-discrimination, other issues are taking precedent; for example, responding to social need, ethnic difference, and the problems associated with HIV/AIDS becoming a chronic condition. This shift has been so dramatic that the work to prevent new infections is being threatened.

This change in perspective can be illustrated by the view of the so-called 'primarily affected groups' which en masse once constituted the heart of AIDS work. Today the picture of gay men, drug users and women is more differentiated. We see that each group is composed of a large variety of subgroups, the experiences of infected persons shaping this awareness of the differences. For example, gay men are today divided into various categories depending on the degree they are affected by the disease. As mentioned above, HIV infection is undergoing a socio-epidemiological shift to marginalised segments of the 'gay community'. (See Bochow, Chapter 12; Marcus, Chapter 3.) With the 'normalisation' of AIDS the typical class-based epidemiological pattern for infectious diseases is being detected in Europe also for HIV, a development already noted several years ago in the USA.

Given this changing view, the responsibility of the AIDS service movement to the so-called 'primarily affected groups' needs to be defined more precisely. This requires:

- Delineating the risk and vulnerability for HIV among the various subgroups of gay men, drug users and women, based on epidemiological data;
- Developing methods of emancipatory health promotion within socially and culturally marginalised populations so as to apply successfully the experience of AIDS prevention to these groups;
- Structuring the services of the ASOs to be responsive to the needs of people with HIV/AIDS from other countries, a heterogeneous group which is likely to grow in the context of inconsistent immigration and asylum policies.

In light of these socio-epidemiological developments the emancipatory basis for AIDS work can also be more precisely defined: we must attempt to promote health through self-help initiatives within the segments of society where there are the most barriers to such structures, namely among the less privileged and among marginalised ethnic groups. This attempt can only succeed if the organised interests of these groups, and not some pure professionalism, is able to define the issues related to AIDS. To the extent to which the institutionalised AIDS service structures are prepared critically to examine their work in light of the political and social interests of the 'primarily affected groups' by reflecting on the interests of people with HIV/AIDS can the ASOs avoid developing a myopic vision which sees only the more privileged members of the groups they are trying to reach. Connecting health promotion to the political interests of the groups to be served reflects a choice to limit voluntarily the scope of health promotion. At the same time, the professional standards of AIDS work serve to guard against the domination of any particular group due to some collective egoism. Not every need formulated by members of an affected group constitutes an imperative for ASOs to act. Not every wish is a command if it stands in contradiction to the established priorities and professional criteria. But the latter are not dogma; they must be flexible and thus capable of achieving balance in difficult circumstances.

To summarise: if the services offered by the ASOs:

- education, outreach-based prevention, and public information
- professional exchange, counselling and self-help-support
- nursing and psychosocial services

are methodologically based on integrating the following:

- prevention at the levels of individual behaviour and the social environment

- primary, secondary and tertiary prevention
- health promotion and self-help

then the goal can be reached of striking a balance between desire and short-term pleasure on the one hand and the need for lasting well-being on the other, at both the individual and collective levels. The extent to which this can be achieved will depend on how well ethical and philosophical issues are reconciled, above all the classical conflict between free-will and happiness and the utopian ideal of a society in which, to use modern terms, self-determination and well-being can co-exist.

Setting limits on the concept of health promotion

To the degree that health promotion is tied to specific values and interests, as described above, can it avoid being confined to a narrow definition of prevention while at the same time relativising its scope. Health is not identical with an all-encompassing state of well-being as suggested by the WHO; that is, it is not a value unto itself. Health is rather a prerequisite for being as free and happy as possible. Indeed health is the goal of all health promotion efforts, but health has its price and sometimes the price is too high. Health is not an end unto itself, but rather it is limited and determined by happiness and free-will as well as by the sense of well-being and the self-determination of the individual. Therefore, within the concept of health promotion itself there is an inherent qualitative limit set on prevention. Not every intervention is justified, even if someone's life or health is at stake. Prevention is about enabling people to weigh risks with the goal of striking their own balance between desire, pleasure and health. Adopting this view early in the movement steered the German ASOs away from the obsession of needing to stop every new infection at all cost.

The self-limiting critical concept of health promotion walks a thin line between the two maxims: living a long life and making life worth living (in German: *dem Leben Jahre und den Jahren Leben geben*). From this perspective the argument is unacceptable that interventions to lengthen a person's life are intrinsically incompatible with his or her desire to maximise the quality of life. However, a critical health promotion recognises and respects the fact that people can act contrary to their own interests, whether due to want or excess, intention or whim, weakness or will power, and conscious or unconscious motivation. Particularly marginalised groups, being closer to and more affected by funda-mental social and cultural conflicts, can be expected to be on more shaky ground and thus plagued more by irrationality, ignorance and the abyss of self. By adopting the slogan 'Making life worth living' (in German: *Den Jahren Leben geben*) the Deutsche AIDS-Hilfe shows a self-critical distance to its mandate and thus makes its own interventions to lengthen people's lives answerable to this qualitative criterion.

This brings us to a central issue in any form of health promotion: what does it mean to extend the time of my life or of others' lives? If health is not reduced to a mechanistic concept of unimpeded bodily functioning, one quickly finds that a qualitative element arises as a counterpoint to the quantitative 'value' of time in terms of length of life. This qualitative element is not officially recorded anywhere. All economic and business calculations of health risks and costs are not able to take into account the concrete reality of being confronted with one's own finite life. Time is not measurable by a clock but by one's own bodily growth and decline. Since quality and quantity of time are inseparable, the economic struggle to value time as money fails in the end. From a subjective perspective the balance between immediate gratification and long-term well-being cannot be expressed in dollars and cents, and it thus loses its value. At the same time, the worth of capital evaporates as soon as one is reminded of the finiteness of his/her life. In the banal phrase 'the most important thing is your health' one finds not only a repressive undertone but also an expression of fear on the part of the speaker, the fear of becoming time's fool. It is a fear that one's own plans – one's program for living which started with one's education and will end in retirement – will be disrupted by the unruliness of the body, of sickness, or of death.

Everyone knows that the basis of all life expectancy calculations are statistical probability, assuming that his or her fate will not deviate much from the norm. Health promotion and prevention seek to introduce some amount of planning and foresight into this arena in order to take away the natural and fateful character of health and sickness. In doing so, we not only play on the irrationality of human behaviour but we also poke around in the darkness of an unforeseeable future. Ultimately, the time which one has is not somehow achieved through one's own actions, but rather it occurs. The future approaches us, and not the other way around. This 'residual unpredictability' is not a *quantité négligeable*, but rather the hard limit which all foresight and planning confront. Here as well, the critical practice of health promotion shows its professional ability to set limits, protecting itself from illusions of grandeur which can only lead to failure or repressive measures.

The threatening German phrase *Volksgesundheit*, which can be rendered into English as 'public health', echoes a not yet forgotten past when health was the subject of public interest under the (pre)Nazi regime. An essential principle for a critical public health is therefore the ability to engage in self criticism and the vigilance to regard every tradition of social medicine and public hygiene as a portent of things past. Health promotion should acknowledge this historical warning by assuming an attitude of humility.

References

Adorno, T. W. (1951) *Minima Moralia. Reflexionen aus dem beschädigten Leben*, Frankfurt/Main: Suhrkamp.
WHO (1986) *Ottawa Charter for Health Promotion*, Geneva: World Health Organisation.

8 The German AIDS self-help movement

The history and ongoing role of AIDS-Hilfe

Rainer Schilling

Introduction

When viewed from a distance and in hindsight, the historical events resulting in the development of the public image and the prevention concepts of the Deutsche AIDS Hilfe (DAH), the National German AIDS Organisation, seem straight-forward and inevitable. However, anyone with experience in social movements would surmise that the development of the DAH was anything but predictable. Retrospective views from the inside of an organisation are often prone to a lack of differentiation between the important and the unimportant. For this reason I want to confine myself to a few remarks which seem significant concerning the history and the development of our concept, focusing on what may make us unique as compared to similar organisations in other countries. I have also concentrated on prevention for gay men, which has been the focus of my work in the national office. If through this chapter myths and legends concerning the Deutsche AIDS-Hilfe are dispelled, I will have fulfilled one of my intentions.

The founding of the Deutsche AIDS-Hilfe (DAH)

Initial news of a mysterious disease concerning gay men appeared in the German press in 1982. West German and West Berlin gays who had American friends or who made trips to the US reported this sickness appearing in the community, first in the leather scene.[1] A concern among organised gay leather men arose that this illness, first called GRID, later AIDS, would find its way over to Germany. This was, for instance, discussed in a small circle of leather men in West Berlin which was joined by the nurse Sabine Lange, an important person in organising hepatitis B vaccinations in the leather scene. In the winter of 1982–3 some men who were working for the Bruno Gmünder gay publishing house joined this circle. These men belonged to the bourgeois, liberal wing of the gay movement. One of them came from Cologne, another one, myself, came from Munich. The discussion about the disease and its possible consequences had already commenced in these two cities.

In contrast to the left-wing, student-influenced gay movement these men were not of the opinion that the virus was an invention of the CIA or somehow a pretext to discriminate against gays. For us it was a real sickness which threatened gay men and their way of life and which ultimately could be used to intensify anti-gay discrimination. Therefore, three questions were intensively discussed in West Berlin that winter:

• How could we establish an independent information service about the new disease which would spread the reports from the US as fast as possible?

• What could we do to ensure that gay German men who had fallen ill would get the best possible professional help and support from the community?

• How could we effectively work against the repression of gays that was to be expected?

It was evident that money would be needed to carry out any plan of action. To be able to acquire donations we decided to set up a non-profit entity. During the initial organisational discussions in Cologne, Munich and Berlin, the circle of 'founding fathers' was enlarged. In Berlin, some gay men with a background in social politics – but without a connection to the leather scene – joined in. In the end the Deutsche AIDS-Hilfe (literally 'German AIDS Assistance') was founded in September 1983 (responsible for Berlin), the Münchener AIDS-Hilfe in January 1984 (for Munich), and the Deutsche AIDS-Hilfe Köln (for Cologne) in the summer of 1984.

Very soon thereafter the Deutsche AIDS-Hilfe had the ambition to become active on a nationwide basis. But only after the Berliner AIDS-Hilfe (in Berlin) was founded as the direct service arm of the Deutsche AIDS-Hilfe, was the idea of a national AIDS umbrella organisation for Germany intensively pursued. During 1985 the Deutsche AIDS-Hilfe went from being a regional organisation serving Berlin to becoming the headquarters for the national federation, comprising all fifteen of the local AIDS organisations which had been founded over the previous two years. The fact that this all occurred so quickly, in contrast to the drawn-out initial phases of the organising process, is most of all due to the political farsightedness, power of conviction, and the lobby work of the second board of directors of the Deutsche AIDS-Hilfe. This board, elected in February 1985 to head the local AIDS service organisation in Berlin, asserted over the course of the following year its position as the leadership of a national organisation. Without this early establishment of an umbrella organisation, the AIDS service movement in Germany would never have been so powerful as it later became. And without an umbrella organisation money would not have been allocated by the Federal Ministry for Health for community-based, nationwide prevention among the most affected groups.

The early years

In January 1986 the staff of the DAH moved into their own office space. Being a national organisation, funds were received from the Federal Ministry for Health to pay for projects and staff. By the end of 1987 more than twenty permanent positions had been created. The last department to be established in 1987 was the Department for Gay Men with myself as one of the personnel. Prior to this, the Department for Drugs and Prisons and the Department for Female and Male Prostitution had been set up. In the beginning of 1988 the Department for People with HIV and AIDS followed.

The Deutsche AIDS-Hilfe was founded by gay men (and one woman) who saw their way of life threatened by a new disease and subsequent repression. In this respect it was a gay self-help group. AIDS prevention could not be considered until HIV was discovered to be the cause of AIDS. With the inclusion of intravenous drug users and prostitutes, as reflected in the composition of the departments at the national office, the DAH became a self-help organisation for all people in the groups in Germany who were primarily at risk for AIDS. These groups were defined by the DAH in a memorandum issued in June 1987.

Having the Department for People with HIV and AIDS made the DAH stand out in a positive way, as compared to similar national institutions in other countries at the time which saw themselves as being only responsible for primary prevention (the preventing of new infections). The inclusion of this department reflected our concept of self-help which included those who were actually affected by HIV and AIDS, the people who were the reason for setting up our organisation in the first place. I also want to mention here that the character and content of our prevention messages has been greatly influenced by the integral role of people with HIV/AIDS in the organisation. For instance, we have always been very careful not to place blame on individuals if they do not practise safer sex or if they do not always engage in safer behaviour.

One can truly say that the 'house' Deutsche AIDS-Hilfe was well furnished in a very short time. But it also made a good impression from the exterior. The DAH indisputably had the leadership position in opinion-making concerning AIDS as well as political weight and a strong reputation in the country.

Of course it was of great advantage that on the political level – thanks to the Minister for Health, Rita Süssmuth – a prevention approach caught on which was based on an individual learning strategy instead of the classical repressive control measures which were being advocated by Peter Gauweiler in Bavaria. (See Frankenberg and Hanebeck, Chapter 4.) The DAH, being a self-help organisation under whose umbrella those at risk for and directly affected by AIDS gathered, was an ideal body for this kind of prevention policy.

An important though controversial strategic position was taken by the DAH – to the annoyance of many physicians – when the HIV antibody test (then the ELISA test) was discussed in the autumn of 1984. At the time, the test was being heralded by the medical community as not only a means of detection but as a means of prevention for HIV. The DAH strongly repudiated this idea, publicly denouncing the test as being unsuitable for this purpose, given that the test itself did not prevent transmission of the virus. Knowing that one was positive did not necessarily mean that you protected others. At that time, the means of transmission were also still unclear. In any case, a positive test resulted in uncertainty and a fear of dying of an untreatable disease while suffering discrimination. In addition, the test result had no medical consequences, as no treatments were then available. Another argument concerned the danger that all responsibility for prevention of the disease would be placed on the shoulders of those who were HIV-positive. For these reasons, the test was seen by the DAH as being an inappropriate method for primary prevention. (See also Rosenbrock, Chapter 19; Frankenberg and Hanebeck, Chapter 4.)

The DAH took another important stand with the already mentioned memorandum of 1987. Under the slogan 'AIDS Concerns Everyone' (*AIDS geht uns alle an*) the Government attempted to reconcile various segments of the general population with the groups of persons most affected by the disease. This slogan was misinterpreted as being a sweeping and undifferentiated appeal for prevention aimed at everybody, the campaign being criticised for implying that all 60 million West Germans had the same risk of infection and thus the same need to be educated.[2] The DAH's memorandum pioneered a more realistic point of view by naming and describing the very differentiated infection risks which do not affect everyone in the same way. This included describing the needs of the groups which were, based on epidemiological data, the most vulnerable at that time and which were thus the groups with the highest need for targeted education. Specifically, the populations designated as target groups were: homosexual men, intravenous drug users, prison inmates and prostitutes. Prostitutes, unlike the other three target groups, were not disproportionately infected with HIV, but they were included nevertheless because of the inherent risk of infection found in their line of work.

Through this memorandum the DAH had a calming effect on hysterical tendencies in the population. At the same time, the naming of the target groups riled some gay activists who feared that the description of gay men as being one of the primarily affected groups would lead to stigmatisation. They feared, not without good reason, that the equating of gay with AIDS would provide support for arguments that the cause for the disproportionate infection rate in this group was the 'gay lifestyle'. The slogan 'Promiscuity is the motor of the epidemic' was indeed already in common use.

It was only with great difficulty that the staff of the DAH's Department for Gay Men in 1988 could defend their intention to be truthful and honest about the disease without playing into the hands of opponents to the gay movement. It was clear to the Department that all forms of blame placed on individuals on the basis of epidemiological data must be fought energetically. The same went for the condemnation of gay lifestyles which was often a topic when such data were presented.

Other opponents of this unequivocal orientation toward the primarily affected groups feared that the image of the DAH and of the local AIDS-Hilfe organisations could be tarnished by this position. This opinion was held mainly by gay men who saw themselves being accepted by society for the first time because of their (charitable) work in the AIDS-Hilfe groups. In spite of all opposition, the central tenet that the DAH should focus on specific target groups was ardently defended by the Department for Gay Men.

Prevention is more than promoting safer sex

More difficult for the Department for Gay Men was another position taken in the same memorandum:

> As a medical solution to the problem is not in sight, the focus of the fight against AIDS clearly must be prevention through education and information. Prevention mainly means motivating the primarily affected groups to learn low risk behaviour patterns in the interest of long-term behavioural change.
> (Memorandum: 9)

The print media that were produced by the DAH when this memorandum was issued show what was meant at the time by 'education and information'. There were leaflets about the use of condoms, several posters whose subject was the means of transmission and the condom, and a leaflet based on one from the US listing sexual practices that were assigned to a scale ranging from safe to unsafe. However, neither the meaning of sexuality nor the negative psychological and emotional consequences of condom use were discussed. We considered this approach to be too reductivist, as it focused solely on factual information about the virus. In our opinion, these early materials were based on a naive educational method which we could not accept, given our knowledge of gay men's sexual experience, based on our work as volunteers in the community.

Even the first poster by the DAH in the summer of 1985 depicting the slogan 'Surely better – safer sex' had a tenor which did not suit us. Our experience in the gay scene told us that safer sex was not better; it was rather viewed as a necessary evil, a disruptive factor which gay men could not and did not want to adopt for every sexual contact. Safer sex simply was not 'better' sex for most gay men. In other words: the concept of prevention which had been developed up to that point in time was based on a rational and cognitive point of view, far removed from a realistic assessment of men's sexual needs.

It was very important for the Department to expand and modify the existing approach toward prevention, placing a greater emphasis on the specific concerns raised by the primarily affected groups. For that purpose, we not only brought together the experiences of West German outreach workers and the opinions of leading German psychologists and sexual scientists, but we also critically examined international concepts for prevention which were available at the time. The WHO Ottawa Charter concerning health promotion (WHO, 1986) soon became a fundamental part of the prevention concept for the Department, given the Charter's emphasis on lifestyle and health.

The outcome of the process to define the basis for prevention work was the white paper 'Gay Men and AIDS' which was composed during a meeting in May 1989 and was passed by the members of the DAH general assembly in the same year. This paper states the core principles which are valid to this day for the preventative work among gay men. For that reason, I would like to quote the essential passages from the third chapter, thus documenting here that the DAH took a stand early in its history which was only later adopted on an international basis, and which is still controversial in some countries:

> The DAH supports the definition of health as proposed by the WHO. Health is not limited to the mere absence of sickness or symptoms of disease. Health is a condition of physical, psychological, spiritual, and social well-being. Prevention can not confine itself to medical interventions for individuals but must, in this holistic understanding of health, consider all spheres of life and their pathological effects.
>
> Prevention for the DAH is not limited to specific behaviours on the part of the individual to avoid HIV infection. Prevention goes beyond safer sex campaigns to include:
> * the support of self-acceptance and self-confidence
> * the promotion of divergent lifestyles to be accepted by society at large
> * the dismantling and deterrence of discrimination
> * the promotion of the ability to exercise responsibility for one's self and one's actions
> * the promotion, protection, and development of sexuality in its many forms.
>
> [. . .]
>
> The primary aim of prevention work is to enable the individual to make choices (i.e., promoting the individual capacity to act). This aim can only be reached through a process of changing individual and collective factors and by exerting influence on the social environment.
>
> [. . .]
>
> The decision for or against safer sex is the decision of an individual for or against the reduction of infection risk. This decision is not made once and for all, but must be considered in each new situation. This decision is dependent on a variety of factors and conditions; e.g., the degree of self-acceptance, the characteristics of the situation itself, the desire for security, and the desire for intimacy with another human being.

In this position paper we intentionally did not distinguish between prevention which focuses on behaviours and prevention which focuses on the social environment (*Verhaltens- und Verhältnisprävention*) because the individual is at the centre of our work. Our goal is changing an individual's behaviour, but this behaviour is intrinsically connected to the environment in which it is performed. We wanted to change the social conditions in which the individual lives so as to enable him/her to change his/her behaviour, to make it possible for him/her to act in a competent way. Unifying prevention which focuses on behaviour with prevention which focuses on the social environment is the central theme of the white paper, a theme which later became a cornerstone of the prevention concept of the DAH. This concept was defined from 1991 onward as *structural prevention*. (See Etgeton, Chapter 7, for a more thorough discussion of this concept.)

With the white paper we wanted to show the limits of rational, cognitive-based education without disputing its necessity. We view strengthening self-esteem and personal identity to be at least as equally important as imparting information. We summarised this position using the following statement. 'Emancipation is prevention'. This does not mean, however, that prevention is necessarily emancipating. The latter would mean that factual information about transmission, an important element of HIV prevention, necessarily leads to emancipation. This is, of course, not the case. (See Etgeton, Chapter 7.)

In our white paper it was also important for us to present arguments for the preservation and expansion of gay community structures, going beyond instrumentalising these structures for safer sex campaigns. At the same time, we wanted to explain why it is important to use specific (and often explicit) language or depictions regarding sex when trying to reach the target groups. In our view, use of this language was an expression of a broader prevention concept and not simply a tool of public relations or social marketing. As another passage from the white paper makes clear:

> Communicating the acceptance of a lifestyle in both language and images is not only done in order to reach the target audience with our safer sex message or to become more credible as an AIDS service organisation. In addition, we want to promote the individual and collective emancipation process, including the power of self-determination.

> We do not want to infringe upon gay communication structures and venues. Through such infringement, we not only could compromise our ability to bring our prevention message across, but also we could potentially cause damage to these locations as places of learning and as places which are indispensable for gay identity and emancipation.

In light of the limits of fact-based rational models for education, the Department for Gay Men of the DAH carried out training sessions for outreach workers, gay bar owners, and coming out group leaders. The Department has tried ever since to promote the practice of safer sex in the different subgroups, including young men coming out, through the use of brochures and other media. This has included the distribution of matchbooks, postcards, coasters, ball point pens, and other give-aways showing reminders of safer sex practices. In all of the various campaigns, the DAH has depicted gay lifestyles positively while promoting solidarity between the various scenes and persons with HIV and AIDS.

Of course the images used have changed over time and the copy and topics have become more differentiated. Nevertheless we continue to concentrate on supporting identity formation and strengthening self-esteem through counteracting internalised feelings of shame and guilt. Over time we have taken up topics directed to new subgroups which we had not included previously. Gay leather men was the first group to receive such attention. Later came bisexual and hearing-impaired men. Specific situations have also found a place in our prevention efforts. For example, gay men on holiday as well as men in relationships. Regarding the latter, we have sought to bring the so-called 'risk factor love' to the attention of the target group (see Dannecker, Chapter 11). In recent years, we have also expanded the scope of our materials to include information about other sexually transmitted diseases, including especially hepatitis.

Looking toward the future: identifying vulnerable populations

The stable number of new infections through homosexual transmission in Germany speaks for the success of our work. (See Marcus, Chapter 3.) We have never given in to the illusion that we could avoid each and every new infection. We now know, however, that the new infections happen increasingly in those groups that are socially or culturally at a disadvantage and who therefore are less able to act preventively. These groups include homosexually-active working class men, immigrants, and male prostitutes (hustlers). (See Marcus, Chapter 3; Bochow, Chapter 12.)

We are still in the early stages of developing effective prevention for these populations. According to the principle of structural prevention, this work must go beyond the transmission of knowledge about HIV. A central problem is that we do not yet know how to strengthen personal identity in these groups nor how to enable them to take action in protecting their health. Another reason for the lack of effective prevention is the limited potential for self-help in these populations, particularly as compared to gay middle class men. Finally, the middle class background of both paid and voluntary staff of the local AIDS service organisations presents a barrier to reaching these groups, impeding the development of appropriate communication models and the initiative to make contact to the groups in the first place. We are also at the early stages of designing suitable prevention strategies for gay men from the former East Germany, strange as this may seem. For far too long the East was inundated with concepts based on West German socialisation and constructs of homosexuality, without any resistance being expressed by colleagues and target groups in that part of the country. (See Herrn, Chapter 13.)

AIDS is on its way to becoming a chronic, treatable – if not curable – disease. The intense fear of dying once experienced by the newly infected has abated. The new combination therapies have, at least for the moment, shown unexpected success. AIDS is becoming something banal, losing its previous drama. However, through this 'normalisation' stable safer sex behaviour over a long period of time is becoming more difficult, especially in those groups for whom health is not considered to be a major priority and who have little control in shaping their own lives, for instance the working class. The DAH will nevertheless leave no stone unturned to find ways of promoting an awareness of health issues among all target groups, an awareness which is not focused on a fear of death but rather on the conviction that even 'normal' diseases are avoidable.

We are aware that this task is difficult, not the least because there is another side to the 'normalisation' of AIDS: AIDS is no longer a topic in the media and is disappearing from the minds of those who have up to now politically and financially supported the AIDS service organisations. The willingness to volunteer for AIDS work is also diminishing as seen in the dwindling numbers of volunteers in the gay community, even though AIDS is still with us. We have our work cut out for us in the years to come.

Notes

1   The so-called 'leather scene' is a segment of the gay community in many countries which is organised into local, national and international clubs, and which operates its own commercial establishments ('leather bars'). Many of these men have a preference for leather clothing and paraphernalia, hence the name.
2   The reader is reminded that Germany was divided until the Wall fell in 1989. The Deutsche AIDS-Hilfe was, therefore, an exclusively West German organisation until reunification. See Herrn, Chapter 13, for a description of prevention in East Germany during the early years of the epidemic.

References

WHO (1986) *Ottawa Charter for Health Promotion*, Geneva: World Health Organisation.

Part III
Risk perception and decision making in safer sex

9 Reactions of the general population to AIDS

The relationship between sociodemographic variables and lay concepts of disease aetiology

Rüdiger Jacob, Willy H. Eirmbter and Alois Hahn

AIDS: the starting point

In Germany the prevalence of HIV is still low, compared to other diseases, but AIDS remains one of the main causes of death for young adults (Heilig, 1989). Although the virus is difficult to transmit and is directly connected to very specific behaviours, AIDS has caused social reactions like stigma and exclusion of infected persons and persons believed to be infected, reactions which are not commensurate with the actual threat posed by the disease. For that reason, the term 'social infection with AIDS' (Bleibtreu-Ehrenberg, 1987) was coined to describe the reaction of society to the epidemic.

It is obvious that the general public has many ways of acknowledging and interpreting AIDS and that these various reactions can diverge from the 'correct' view as propagated by science and by public health information campaigns. Subjective explanations for events, so-called everyday theories, are much more relevant for determining attitude and behaviour than 'objective' facts because they offer an immediate sense of security which serves as a basis for orientation and action. (See Laucken, 1974.) Sixty years ago the American social psychologist William Thomas described this phenomenon with his Thomas Theorem, which in its general form states: 'If men [people] define situations as real, they are real in their consequences' (Thomas, 1932: 572).

Lay concepts of disease aetiology

Medicine constitutes a collectively accepted body of knowledge which serves as a basis for our behaviour regarding diseases. We could hypothesize that in modern society the so-called everyday theories regarding sickness and health have become less important, given the influential role of medicine. This is, however, not the case.

Medical terms, like other technical terminology, are not completely adopted into common, everyday ways of thinking; however, the latter also has content which is not found in specialised medical knowledge. This is the case because scientific theories regard diseases and bodily processes isolated from their subjects; the personal meanings which connect the subjective experiences of life and disease are not seen as legitimate areas for medical inquiry. However, the body is not only an object of medical research, it is also the centre of self-interpretation and social orientation. (For a more detailed discussion see Jacob, 1995; Jacob *et al.*, 1997.)

In almost every society there exist patterns of interpretation which see physical malfunction as a sign of hidden truth. Modern biomedical science, with its emphasis on the mechanistic aspects of disease, stands in sharp contrast to these patterns. In many cultures disease is interpreted as disgrace, punishment, or a form of self-disclosure which reveals one's true character. As a result, sickness can present an additional burden to the individual when even minor physical symptoms are interpreted as disclosing certain qualities of the person which are subject to social stigma (Jacob *et al.*, 1997).

Closely associated with stigma is the tendency toward blaming the sick person, a phenomenon which is more intensified when little is known about the disease and when the disease is widespread in a population. Blaming always assumes the aetiology of the disease, thus helping to explain why certain persons are affected. This makes the spread of the disease in a population easier to cope with (Jacob, 1995). In addition, the labelling of certain groups as being responsible for the origin and the spread of a disease offers room for the exercise of collectively therapeutic 'venting customs'. These customs allow for segregation, isolation, or even eradication of the stigmatised guilty groups and therefore a supposed victory over the disease.

Historical epidemiological research demonstrates impressively the existence of strategies and explanations to avoid infection which are based on the theory and culture of everyday life. This phenomenon is especially prominent in times of large epidemics like the plague, cholera, or syphilis (for example, Gouldsblom, 1979; Rouffié and Sournia, 1987).

Recent studies of how people perceive cancer emphasize the importance of lay concepts of disease aetiology and the persistence of these concepts to this day in spite of scientifically-based explanations. The surveys of Dornheim and Verres show that the belief that cancer is infectious (through sexual or even casual physical contact) is particularly prevalent in rural areas, resulting in the avoidance of cancer patients (Dornheim, 1983; Verres, 1986). Often cancer is viewed as being connected with tuberculosis, cholera, smallpox, or the plague. Cancer, although a relatively new epidemic historically, is associated with collective patterns of explanation which were in use even before the occurrence of the disease. It is also interesting that cancer is associated with an 'unhealthy lifestyle' and sexual excess, both of which are the result of culpable behaviour on the part of those affected (Dornheim, 1983; Verres, 1986). In the case of AIDS the connection between disease, morality and guilt is even more pronounced because HIV is truly infectious and it is transmitted primarily through sexual contact.

The social ramifications of these forms of interpretation are always similar, stemming from the same 'solution' to the problem of disease. If the belief is widespread that avoiding infected persons is the only way to escape from disease and death, people will do just that. Our work has revealed that, in the case of AIDS, there are not only explicit wishes for avoiding contact to those infected, but also for excluding infected persons from social contact and for instituting compulsory measures to control their behaviour (Eirmbter *et al.*, 1993; Jacob *et al.*, 1997).

AIDS: how avoidable is the risk?

From a general theoretical point of view, reactions to serious diseases constitute a paradigm for how people behave when confronted with risk, more generally. In principle two types of reactions can be described, based on the degree to which the person believes he or she can influence the risk at hand. There are reactions to risk which is perceived to be outside the control of the individual (uncontrollable risk), and reactions related to risk over which the person believes he or she has some power (controllable risk).[1] When a disease is viewed as a controllable risk, the sickness is attributed to the individual and his/her choices. This form of risk is viewed as being avoidable if one gives up certain behaviours. On the other hand, if a disease is viewed as being the result of an uncontrollable risk, the sickness is attributed to external forces in the environment which are not affected by a person's actions (for example, see Luhmann, 1988; 1990).

For centuries the classic example of uncontrollable risk was serious infectious diseases. One became infected regardless of the choices you made; it seemed to be a matter of fate, especially where little was known about the disease transmission. The only chance to escape an infection was therefore a general avoidance or isolation of sick persons. This view of disease as an uncontrollable risk changed with the advances in medical science. At the same time the notion that individuals could avoid becoming infected through their own actions grew as more information became available about the effects of vaccines, treatment and preventive behaviour (Gouldsblom, 1979).

It is a characteristic of our time to increasingly interpret risks as the result of personal actions, including risks once thought to be uncontrollable. The problem is how to classify a given risk in a given situation:

> That which is a controllable risk for one person can be an uncontrollable risk for someone else. The smoker risks cancer through his/her own behaviour, but endangers others who are not choosing to take this risk. The same is true for the driver who recklessly passes someone on the highway, the designers and the operators of nuclear power stations, as well as for genetic engineers.
> (Luhmann, 1986: 88)

The case of AIDS provides a good example of the difficulty in interpreting a risk phenomenon as being controllable or uncontrollable. Initially, there was tremendous uncertainty in the general population due to a lack of knowledge and widespread speculation. This new disease fulfilled all the conditions necessary to be subsumed into the traditional everyday theoretical patterns of interpretation of serious diseases: it remains unclear why certain infected people develop AIDS; until recently there have been no reliable therapies; and the disease makes no distinction between young and old, rich or poor. In this sense, AIDS has appeared to be an uncontrollable risk.

On the other hand AIDS, in contrast to past epidemics, is not ubiquitous nor easily transmitted. Not everybody is at equal risk of infection because HIV transmission is restricted to specific behaviours under the control of the individual. The avoidance of an infection can be managed by observing safety measures or by avoiding risk situations altogether. Therefore, AIDS represents a danger resulting from a controllable risk.

At this point one could argue that this false dualism of controllable versus uncontrollable risk can be easily resolved through providing information to the general population about how the virus is transmitted, based on current medical knowledge. This should, at least theoretically, put to rest the view of HIV infection as being a result of some external force while focusing people's attention on the 'objectively correct' point of view; namely, that HIV transmission is contingent on an individual's actions.

This has, in fact, been the goal of all information campaigns until now. There is one important obstacle, however. It cannot be assumed that the interpretation of AIDS risk is related to any particular situation. Rather, the interpretation of the risk as controllable or uncontrollable may be defined by the person long before the situation arises, thereby determining in advance how he/she will perceive AIDS risk. As Albert Einstein once said 'Our theory determines what we are able to observe'. Therefore, what information is internalised, and in which form, depends less on a person's knowledge about the danger of the moment than on his/her basic patterns of risk interpretation.

The view of AIDS as an uncontrolled risk influences the perception of this disease and leads to the interpretation that HIV is highly infectious and ubiquitous. AIDS is an easy target for projection and blaming, because certain stigmatised groups (homosexuals and drug users) comprise the most affected groups in several Western industrialised countries. Not only persons actually infected by the virus can be subsumed by this dynamic, but also all members of the so-called 'high-risk groups'. In the end, because of the imagined ubiquity of AIDS, all others can indiscriminately be the objects of projection and fear, at least all persons outside the immediate sphere of the individual making the judgement. At the root is the perception that the risk of AIDS originates with others, so it is a risk which lurks everywhere.

It follows from the above that a general mistrust of all strangers is an inherent pre-condition for preventing an infection. Contact with a carrier of the virus has to be avoided because of the imagined danger of transmission. As a result there is a wish for excluding infected persons from everyday life. And since there is no way to regulate all potentially threatening situations (for example, public toilets, visiting a doctor, public transport, etc.) compulsory state-run measures are deemed necessary. In this view, such measures are not regarded as being repressive; it is in the interest of healthy people to require infected persons to undergo certain treatments. It makes no difference whether such measures are presented as therapy (analogous to committing persons with psychiatric illness) or as a deserved punishment (corresponding to the arrest of criminals).

In contrast, the assessment of AIDS as a controllable risk implies a conscious and calculated confrontation with the threat of HIV infection. On the basis of official information, risk situations can simply be avoided. This point of view advocates behaviour appropriate to the risk present in the particular situation as opposed to a general mistrust when in contact with others. The focus is on changing one's own behaviour as a reaction to the potential for infection. The identification and treatment of the carrier of the virus is therefore not necessary, because it is not the infected person her/himself who is threatening, but forms of contact with him or her.

Research questions and hypotheses

The above argument was summarised in the following hypotheses for our research:

- Lay knowledge is more important for behaviour than scientific knowledge about HIV. This is so because lay knowledge, in contrast to scientific knowledge, is more stable over time, is more readily available, and it offers interpretations which give meaning to the disease phenomenon. For these reasons, lay knowledge offers a subjectively more secure foundation for understanding HIV and responding to it, with the perception of the disease and its interpretation not being separable from each other.
- The importance of lay concepts for cancer is well-researched, pointing to the association between cancer and such diseases as tuberculosis and the plague. These concepts lead to fear of becoming infected with cancer, to avoidance of affected persons, and to blaming cancer patients for the transgressions which led to their being punished by disease. A lay concept of cancer is associated with an 'unhealthy lifestyle' and sexual excesses.
- In the case of AIDS the fear of infection and the relationship between disease, morality and blame is even more important because AIDS is transmitted through sexual contacts. In addition, homosexuals were the group in Western industrial countries who were affected first. The problem with scientific knowledge from the standpoint of the average person is that it does not fulfill expectations of reliability, longevity or truth because of its rules of accumulation and refutation. Scientific theories, including theories of medicine, have often been proven wrong. For that reason, it is comprehensible why scientific knowledge and recommendations are not necessarily adopted by everyday theories related to behaviour. The lay person can argue that what science says today is harmless (for example, casual contact) may turn out to be dangerous tomorrow on the basis of new findings.
- There are two primary modes of assessing AIDS risk which have different behavioural consequences. In the first case, AIDS is regarded as a

controllable risk based on the official information campaigns. People can protect themselves through monitoring their own behaviour. One needs to avoid certain situations, but there is no cause for stigma or avoidance regarding infected persons. In the second case, AIDS is regarded as a highly infectious disease, with some believing it is as contagious as the common cold. AIDS is an uncontrollable risk which cannot be prevented through measures taken by the individual, with the exception of avoiding and excluding infected or sick persons.

• We can assume that the mode of dealing with risk has a particular social distribution. A sense of security and self-confidence as well as the readiness to take risk and to tackle various problems are functions of specific life circumstances, personal histories and socialisation processes. Socio-economic status (as a function of education and job status), age and the social environment are important indicators. It is likely that a younger age, higher socio-economic status, and living in an urban environment are associated with an enhanced ability to adapt and respond to HIV. Therefore, it is expected that younger, better educated and professionally successful city dwellers will be more likely to view AIDS as a controllable risk. Whereas, older people who live in the country or in small towns with a lower socio-economic status will be more likely to see AIDS as an uncontrollable risk.

We formulated the following research questions based on the above hypotheses:

• What ideas about AIDS, what fears concerning infection, and what behavioural reactions to the disease are found in the general public? We summarised this question by asking: What dispositions are present in the population regarding AIDS?
• Does the content of a particular disposition correspond to specific lay theories?
• Does each disposition have a particular social distribution?

Methodology

A total of three population-based surveys were conducted. In the summer of 1990, 2,118 people were randomly sampled from the then West Germany. In the winter of 1991–2, an additional 2,132 persons were sampled in the then East Germany. Both samples were administered the same standardised questionnaire. For Germany as a whole a replication of the survey was performed in the summer of 1995; it is the results of this last wave which will be presented here. The questionnaire was part of the ZUMA Social Science Survey (*ZUMA – Sozialwissenschaften – BUS*). This national survey is conducted several times a year in Germany, covering a variety of topics. The survey is organised by the Centre for Surveys, Methods and Analysis (ZUMA, Mannheim). GFM/GETAS (Hamburg) was in charge of the fieldwork.

The population sampled was adults residing in Germany, with subjects being interviewed in their homes. Subjects were selected using the ADM Master Samples, a multi-stage and stratified random sample.

The total sample of the survey in 1995 was 5,040; 3,360 from the former West Germany and 1,680 from the former East Germany. The adjusted random sample (after removing cases with quality-neutral and systematic missing responses) contained 3,156 cases. This adjusted sample was included in the analysis. In total there were 2,077 cases from the former West Germany and 1,079 cases from the former East Germany. The response rate was 67.8 per cent for western Germany and 70.1 per cent for the eastern part of the country. ZUMA wanted a disproportionate East/West stratification in the sample so as to have a broad basis for a special analysis of the eastern German data. For analysis of the data set as a whole, however, a weighting procedure was employed to address this over-representation. More details about the methodology of the survey can be found in Eirmbter *et al.* (1993); Hahn *et al.* (1996); and Jacob *et al.* (1997).

Selected results

Through a correspondence analysis the data was tested for the hypothesised characteristics of persons exhibiting the two dispositions toward AIDS risk.[2] These two dispositions are: AIDS perceived as an uncontrollable risk and AIDS perceived as a controllable risk.[3] Theoretically a two-dimensional solution for the analysis is possible, given the three response categories of the dependent variable. That is, it should be possible to detect the factors associated both with the perception of AIDS as an uncontrollable risk and with the perception of AIDS as a controllable risk. However, since the first axis (AIDS as an uncontrollable risk) alone describes 94.1 per cent of the variance, only the results associated with this axis are presented here (a more detailed description of variable definition and analytic method can be found in Jacob *et al.*, 1997).

The dependent variable was entered into the analysis with eighteen independent variables, essentially operationalising the sociodemographic characteristics associated with disease perception, as discussed above. The correspondence analysis allowed us to determine which of the independent variables cluster around the two forms of perceived AIDS risk, or in terms of the statistical procedure, around the two axes of the dependent variable. The results of the analysis are presented in Table 9.1.

A correspondence analysis allows for the simultaneous analysis of both the rows and columns in a contingency table. Analogous to a principle components analysis (used for continuous data), row and column profiles (that is, the row and column proportions for each cell, adjusted by the marginal totals) are projected onto non-correlated axes representing dimensions. The table shown here uses the terminology generated by the SIMCA program, designating the inertia and coefficient values obtained. The procedure involves weighting the individual row and column profiles by their inertia or 'mass,' which designates

Table 9.1 Results of the correspondence analysis for AIDS perceived as an uncontrollable risk

Dependent variable	Abbrev.	Mass	Loc1	Sqcor1	Ctr1
AIDS as an uncontrollable risk					
agreement	g1	72	517	912	364
neither agree nor disagree	g2	289	237	924	306
disagreement	g3	639	-166	994	331
Associated characteristics					
Region					
West	W	38	1	1	0
East	E	20	6	14	0
Age					
18–29		18	10	-141	995	4 ←
30–39		30	12	-153	1,000	5 ←
40–49		40	9	50	981	0
50–59		50	10	23	402	0
60+		60	17	163	985	8 ←
Education					
None	KA	2	364	923	6 ←
Primary school diploma	HS	24	167	1000	13 ←
Tenth grade diploma	MR	19	-41	877	1
College preparation/college	AB	12	-327	981	23 ←
Population of city/town					
under 5,000	DO	11	52	925	1
5,000–50,000	KS	22	48	606	1
50–100,000	MS	4	53	1000	0
over 100,000	GS	20	-85	770	3
Religiosity					
very	sF	13	71	533	1
somewhat	mF	20	18	535	0
not religious	nF	6	-26	157	0
Infection through casual contact					
0	k0	20	-340	994	43 ←
1	k1	9	-220	943	8
2	k2	8	41	115	0
3	k3	7	121	913	2 ←
4+	k4	14	579	997	89 ←
Infected persons are to blame					
agree	s1	19	394	999	55 ←
neither agree nor disagree	s2	19	75	420	2
disagree	s3	19	-449	960	73 ←
Infected persons should be excluded					
agree	a1	10	797	909	124 ←
neither agree nor disagree	a2	19	192	537	13 ←
disagree	a3	28	-414	997	91 ←

Table 9.1 (continued)

Associated Characteristics	Abbrev.	Mass	Loc1	Sqcor1	Ctr1
Acceptance of compulsory measures					
0	z0	12	-408	991	37 ←
1	z1	10	-276	996	14 ←
2	z2	11	-76	663	1
3	z3	10	184	1000	7 ←
4 or 5	z4	15	452	999	57 ←
Threatened by technology					
very	t1	46	-4	95	0
somewhat	t2	10	-11	35	0
not threatened	t3	1	602	988	6 ←
Scepticism with regard to the medical system					
agree	m1	17	174	927	10 ←
neither agree nor disagree	m2	29	31	353	1
disagree	m3	11	-341	995	24 ←
Internal locus of control					
agree	i1	40	-81	986	5 ←
neither agree nor disagree	12	13	121	956	3
disagree	13	1	378	986	3
External locus of control					
agree	e1	10	416	822	32 ←
neither agree nor disagree	e2	26	6	6	0
disagree	e3	19	-292	998	30 ←
Threatened by infectious diseases					
very	p1	15	393	990	43 ←
somewhat	p2	28	-82	853	4
not threatened	p3	14	-238	995	15 ←
Threatened by chronic diseases					
very	c1	30	87	960	4
somewhat	c2	20	-79	997	2
not threatened	c3	7	-102	826	1
Infectivity of cancer					
very	kk	2	674	962	18 ←
somewhat	kw	7	516	917	33 ←
not infectious	kn	45	-133	964	15 ←
Infectivity of AIDS					
very	ak	30	135	959	10 ←
somewhat	aw	19	-206	952	15 ←
not infectious	an	6	-167	916	3
Threatened in the public sphere					
0 or 1	o1	7	-209	942	6 ←
2	o2	7	-247	983	8 ←
3	o3	20	-82	622	2
4 or 5	o4	22	242	989	24 ←

Note: The arrows designate characteristics of particular importance for the dependent variable.

the relative contribution of the characteristic represented. 'Loc' means Location, that is the position of the characteristic on the corresponding axis. The 'Contribution' (Ctr) for each axis is a measure of how strongly the characteristic contributes to the axis. Contribution is a function of mass and distance from the origin, which one can imagine as a balance beam. This means that profiles with lower mass scores will have higher contribution scores and therefore they are particularly important in defining the axis, the further they are from the origin. The interpretation of the coefficients need to take into account the other contribution coefficients of the model for the particular dimension (rule of thumb: the larger the coefficient, the stronger the influence the characteristic has on the axis). In other words: the contribution (Ctr) is a measure for the degree to which the axis is explained by the particular variable. 'QCor' designates the quadratic correlation of the characteristic with the axis, corresponding to the factor loading of the factor analysis procedure. QCor is, therefore, a measure for explaining how much variance of the characteristic is explained by the axis. (See Blasius, 1988; Greenacre, 1984.)

The results of our analysis suggest that the disposition toward AIDS as an uncontrollable risk is most likely to be found among persons who possess several characteristics. Older persons with a lower level of education and residing in a rural area or small town would tend to view AIDS in this way. Whether a person lives in eastern or western Germany appears, however, not to have an influence, with the view of AIDS as an uncontrollable risk found in both parts of the country. Blaming persons infected or thought to be infected with HIV is also characteristic of this view of AIDS, with 'different' and 'strange' minority groups seen as threats to the subject's values and norms. Accordingly the willingness for avoiding affected persons and the acceptance of compulsory measures for the protection of the public's health are also present.

The view of AIDS as an uncontrollable risk is also associated with various fears, including the fear of infectious diseases in general and the fear of becoming infected with HIV through casual contact. The fear of chronic, degenerative disease may be a function of age, because older people are more affected by such conditions. This could explain the presence of this variable within the cluster of characteristics. However, a pronounced belief in the infectiousness of cancer points to a more generalised fear of disease transmission of various kinds. The heightened perceived threat of infectious diseases among these subjects supports this impression of a generalised fear, because such diseases have little relevance for mortality and morbidity in Germany. The mistrust of the health system as well as a fear of modern technology are also distinct characteristics of persons viewing AIDS risk as being uncontrollable. A high level of fear is even evident in everyday public situations, subjects feeling threatened due to the potential of crime. Finally, these persons assess their ability to respond effectively to situations as low, as seen in the tendency toward an external versus an internal locus of control.

Discussion

Results show that indeed lay knowledge is more important for behaviour than scientific knowledge about HIV. Similar to cancer, many people associate AIDS with sexual excess and sexual deviation and tend to blame those already ill, especially if they belong to so called 'high-risk-groups'. These people often assess AIDS as an highly infectious disease that can not be controlled by individual behaviour.

The dominance of insecurity and danger in this point of view is understandable when you consider the potential resources and the life experiences of the persons described by the cluster of characteristics resulting from the analysis. We are essentially describing the reactions of older people from age cohorts from the Second World War and the post-war period. Some of these subjects may have also experienced the difficult pre-war period, including the Depression. This age group did not have the resources to improve their situation. It is therefore not surprising that they feel unable to influence risk, having internalised a confusing outer environment into a world-view which sees fate as determining the outcome of events.

In direct contrast to the above group, those who experience AIDS as a controllable risk have very different characteristics. These subjects are younger, better educated, and tend to be from urban centres. AIDS is seen by them as being less infectious, in line with the message of public information campaigns. Casual contact is also not seen as presenting a danger. The willingness to blame people with AIDS for their disease, to exclude infected persons from society, and to institute compulsory control measures are also less pronounced. Infectious diseases are also not regarded as a threat and cancer is not viewed as being infectious. In addition, the health system has positive associations. People of this group also tend to have a high assessment of their ability to take action in situations, being more likely to exhibit an internal versus an external locus of control.

Conclusion

How people perceive and interpret AIDS risk can be traced to particular sociodemographic characteristics. Younger people having grown up in the stable post-war period without material need. In addition, better educated, professionally established persons have no reason to wrangle with questions of fate or to adopt a pessimistic or fatalistic world-view.

Our work reflects the observation of Karl Marx (now somewhat out of fashion) who claimed that being affects consciousness. Our findings support the long-held position that nothing prevents social problems better than improving the living conditions of deprived groups in society: whether the social problem be xenophobia, stigma, or the discrimination of minority groups. Such a position may no longer be popular in a time of fiscal restraint due to a supposed or real lack of resources. But one must question whether it is more costly to address the consequences of social problems or invest in their prevention in the first place. In this sense any prevention campaign, including those focusing on AIDS, have to be part of a larger political strategy to improve living conditions, employment opportunities and the social structure in society.

Notes

1   In the original German version of the manuscript, the distinction between these two forms of risk is made by using the terminology of Luhmann. A *Gefahr* (danger) in German implies a risk over which the person cannot exercise control; whereas a *Risiko* (risk) can be influenced by the individual.

2   In general, correspondence analysis is useful for the uncovering of complex patterns and differences between groups, as in the present case. It is a method of exploration which makes the simultaneous analysis of column and rows in a contigency table possible. Typically, the column represents the dependent variable. There are no restrictions with regard to the level of measurement, an advantage of this method, therefore allowing for the inclusion of nominal data. For a more detailed description see Blasius, 1988 and Greenacre, 1984.

3   The dependent variable is a construct created from an index of 5-point Likert scaled items (for example, 'The risk for AIDS is lurking everywhere' and 'If you really think about it, there is no effective protection against AIDS'). The final form of the index was established through a factor analysis (PCA, Varimax), with all items having a loading factor higher than five being included. For the correspondence analysis, the 5-point scale was collapsed to three categories resulting in: 'agree', 'neither agree nor disagree', 'disagree'. Agreement indicates that AIDS is perceived to be an uncontrollable risk; disagreement indicates that AIDS is perceived to be a controllable risk.

References

Blasius, J. (1988) 'Zur Stabilität von Ergebnissen bei der Korrespondenzanalyse', *ZA-Informationen* 23: 47–62.

Bleibtreu-Ehrenberg, G (1987) 'Fragen Viren nach Moral?' in: S.R. Dunde (ed.) *AIDS – Was eine Krankheit verändert*, Frankfurt/Main: Fischer-Taschenbuch-Verlag: 45–71.

Dornheim, J. (1983) *Kranksein im dörflichen Alltag. Soziokulturelle Aspekte des Umgangs mit Krebs*, Tübingen: Selbstverlag.

Eirmbter, W. H., Hahn, A. and Jacob, R. (1993) *AIDS und die gesellschaftlichen Folgen*, Frankfurt/Main: Campus.

Gouldsblom, J. (1979) 'Zivilisation, Ansteckungsangst, Hygiene' in P. Gleichmann (ed.), *Materialien zu Norbert Elias' Zivilisationstheorie*, Frankfurt/Main: Suhrkamp: 215–52.

Greenacre, M. (1984) *Theory and Applications of Correspondence Analysis,* London: Academic Press.

Hahn, A., Eirmbter, W. H. and Jacob, R. (1996) *AIDS: Krankheitsvorstellungen in Deutschland*, Opladen: Westdeutscher Verlag.

Heilig, G. K. (1989) 'Gibt es demographische Auswirkungen der AIDS-Epidemie in der Bundesrepublik Deutschland?' *Zeitschrift für Bevölkerungswissenschaft*, 15: 247–70.

Jacob, R. (1995) *Krankheitsbilder und Deutungsmuster. Wissen über Krankheit und dessen Bedeutung für die Praxis*, Opladen: Westdeutscher Verlag.

Jacob, R., Eirmbter, W. H., Hahn, A., Hennes, C. and Lettke, F (1997) *AIDS-Vorstellungen in Deutschland. Stabilität und Wandel*, Berlin: edition sigma.

Laucken, U. (1974) *Naive Verhaltenstheorie*, Stuttgart: Klett.

Luhmann, N. (1986) *Ökologische Kommunikation*, Opladen: Westdeutscher Verlag.

—— (1988) *Die Wirtschaft der Gesellschaft*, Frankfurt/Main: Suhrkamp.

—— (ed.) (1990) *Risiko und Gefahr. Soziologische Aufklärung. Fünf konstitutive Perspektiven*, Opladen: Westdeutscher Verlag: 131–69.

Ruffié, J. and Sourina, J. C. (1987) *Die Seuchen in der Geschichte der Menschheit*, Stuttgart: Klett-Cotta.

Thomas, W. S. (1932) *The Child in America*. New York: Knopf.

Verres, R. (1986) *Krebs und Angst. Subjektive Theorien von Laien über Entstehung, Vorsorge, Früherkennung, Behandlung und die psychosozialen Folgen von Krebserkrankungen*, Berlin: Springer.

10 AIDS prevention as a social systems intervention

Risk-taking in the context of different types of heterosexual partnerships

Heinrich W. Ahlemeyer

Introduction

The social epidemiology of AIDS in Germany shows particular sexual practices, such as unprotected vaginal and anal intercourse, to be among the most important means of HIV transmission (Koch, 1987; Marcus, Chapter 3). One effective form of preventing HIV infections is using condoms. Attempts have been made to increase their use by imparting cognitive knowledge about HIV and safer sex and by motivating individuals to adopt preventive behaviour.

As other chapters in this volume attest, such prevention endeavours have been successful in Germany in two respects: they resulted in a generally improved and an overall high level of knowledge about HIV, related risk behaviour, and methods of protection; and they generated a consensus for the idea of prevention (BZgA, 1994; Pott, Chapter 6). Analyses of the epidemiologically relevant data, however, show that actual heterosexual behaviour has changed little in terms of the integration of protective devices, particularly as compared to the homosexual population. For the most part, sexual contact between men and women continues to be unprotected (Koch, 1994). The conspicuous discrepancy between high levels of information and the widespread intention to perform preventive behaviour on the one hand, and common non-preventive sexual behaviour on the other hand, raises the issue of how to find a basis for prevention policies which transcend individual knowledge and attitudes in order to bring about practical behaviour change. What significance does the heterosexual relationship assume in this context? How can this relationship be conceptualised? What practical consequences can be drawn if HIV risk management in the relationship is seen from a systemic rather than an individualistic point of view? These are the research questions this chapter sets out to address.

Background

In our research we began with the hypothesis that it is not the detached individual, but the intimate dyad, which acts either preventively or non-preventively when faced with the risk of HIV infection. The addressee of any modification in heterosexual behaviour in the interest of prevention is the intimate couple. In whatever manner, it is the participants in an intimate relationship who deal with the risk of an HIV infection. At any point in time, this results in one preventive decision and comes together in one preventive action that is either taken or not. There is no form of HIV risk management in a couple which would not require a minimum of communication and co-ordination. HIV prevention in the form of condom use does not, therefore, take place in the head of particular individuals, but is the result of the communicative interaction between sexual partners who act as participants in their intimate relationship (McKinney and Sprecher, 1991). It is therefore in the relational context where the common decision whether to take preventive action takes place.

The individual participates in the intimate relationship with his/her own knowledge, intentions and attitudes (Gerhards and Schmidt, 1992). Communication and interaction in the intimate dyad constitutes, however, a specific factor and a reality level of its own in generating action. Following sociological systems theory, our research conceptualises the communicative properties of sexual relations as social systems of intimate communication (Luhmann, 1984a). In contrast to other communication systems, such as interactions in a neighbourhood or at work, the distinctive unity of intimate systems lies in their orientation toward a sexual interaction of the participants. Their communicative design is geared toward an integration of the physical-sexual dimension. Distinct from everyday reality, the couple engages in constructing an erotic reality through preparation, implementation, generation of meaning, co-ordination, integration, and promotion of the erotic in the face of competing demands. Intimate systems constitute themselves and continue operating in a social environment that is not a part of them.

Beyond this distinctive unity we hypothesised that four basic types of intimate communication exist: (R) Romantic, (H) Hedonistic, (M) Matrimonial, and (P) Prostitution-based intimate systems.

These intimate systems were expected to differ not only in major dimensions of the communicative process, such as time (when the communication takes place) and medium (semantics and mode of communication), but also in their reaction toward HIV-related risks and preventive practices (Ahlemeyer, 1990). It was hypothesised that all HIV-relevant heterosexual interactions take place in one of these four intimate system types, each system type consisting not of real 'persons', but of selectively reproduced communicative elements. Intimate

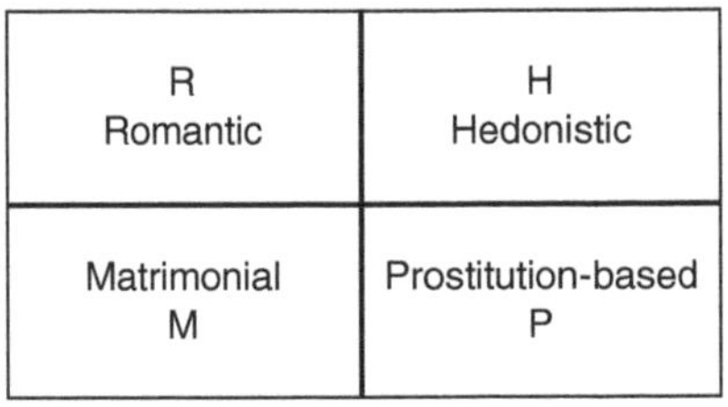

R Romantic	H Hedonistic
Matrimonial M	Prostitution-based P

Figure 10.1 The four basic types of intimate communication systems

systems can be imagined in such a way as to extract from the participants those actions necessary for the ongoing reproduction of the system from moment to moment or, equally, to omit those actions which might endanger or cease a continued system operation (Luhmann, 1984b).

Why propose a systems concept to describe and analyse something as personal as intimate relations? Does the concept of 'the system' not refer to something that is opposed to the private sphere? As contrary as it may be to the thinking of some prevention theorists, the concept of the system lends itself well to an analysis of heterosexual behaviour in the context of HIV risk because it:

1   Allows us to apply the results of modern systems research, in general, as well as sociological systems theory as elaborated by Niklas Luhmann, in particular (Luhmann, 1984b).
2   Facilitates an understanding of both the uniqueness of sexuality and what it has in common with other non-sexual forms of interaction (Weeks, 1986).
3   Provides an adequate theoretical framework to grasp the complexity involved in sexual behaviour (a complexity which comprises altogether different system levels: the organic, the psychological, and the social).
4   Proposes the necessary distinctions for an analytical focus on the social level, which is constituted by communication (Cupach and Metts, 1989).
5   Promotes an appealing intervention philosophy. Contrary to the assumption that a system stands in direct relation to or is somehow directly determined by its environment, the systems approach emphasizes the significance of internal operations within the relationship (Küppers, 1994). In order to relate to their environment, systems first have to organise their own continuity. In searching for ways of improving HIV prevention strategies, it becomes a prerequisite to gain an understanding of the autonomy of sexual communication systems and to analyse more closely what they can actually perceive as useful information (Willke, 1987).

Sample

The sample was taken so as to provide a sufficient number of cases for each of the four basic types of intimate systems (theoretical sampling) and at the same time allow for a wide distribution of participant characteristics – such as age, education, and city/town size – within each of the four intimate systems categories. No claim can be made that the sample is representative, given the sampling method. The participants were recruited mainly through classified ads in diverse print media, but also through contacts to self-help groups and referral by other participants. For the prostitution-based relationships, both prostitutes and clients were directly recruited in red light districts and brothels.

A total of 180 in-depth interviews with men and women from different age groups, educational backgrounds, and cities and towns of various sizes were conducted throughout Germany. Nineteen were excluded from the analysis due to lack of credible self-reporting, competing psychological problems, poor quality of the taped session, missing reports of sexual encounters, etc. Of the remaining 161 interviews, 26 belong to the R Type, 40 to the H Type, 49 to the M Type and 38 to the P Type of relationship, each with an almost equal gender distribution (52.2 per cent female; 48.8 per cent male). There was also an acceptable distribution of other respondent characteristics such as age, education, and size of place of residence. (See Figures 10.2 and 10.3.)

A residual category X contained eight encounters which could not be rated clearly and unambiguously into one of the four basic types. It is this category X in which the diffuse and opaque properties of the intimate systems suggest the gestalt of the fractal. The interviews took place between October 1991 and December 1992. They were conducted according to an interview protocol, with interviewers being prepared for the data-gathering process through extensive training in conducting systemic interviews on sexual behaviour.

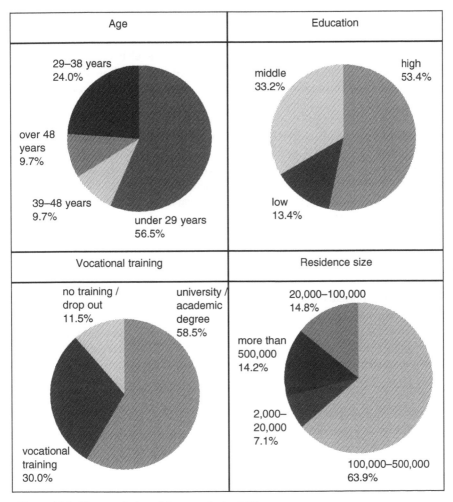

Figure 10.2 Characteristics of the sample (n=161)

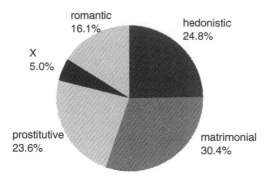

Figure 10.3 Proportion of the sample in each theoretical category of intimate system

Method

Sociocybernetics has assumed a rather mature state in the elaboration of its theoretical basis, in the analysis of sub-system functioning, and in dealing with methodological and epistemological issues.[1] At the same time, it has become indispensable, mostly to psychologists and economists, in specific applications in organisational consulting and family therapy. There is, however, a major gap between theory and praxis which is marked by an almost absent empirical research literature with a systemic orientation (Geyer, 1992). Social science research generally does not use system-oriented approaches, and sociocyberneticists tend to shy away from the hardships of exposing their hypotheses to the examination of social reality.

Formally, the phases of systems-oriented research are no different from any other social science research; namely:

1   the description of the research question
2   the collection of data
3   data analysis
4   and as appropriate concrete recommendations for praxis.

In the course of the research, however, the sociocybernetic approach implies the use of typical systemic approaches in each of these phases, represented here by the acronym ROSI, which stands for:

1   Reframing
2   Observing the system
3   Selecting and distinguishing
4   and Intervening indirectly.

The first three phases were addressed in the portion of the research described here and will be detailed below.

Reframing

Before any social problem can be analysed systemically, it has to be re-conceptualised in sociocybernetic terms. The first step is to clarify the underlying problem: whose problem is it and why is it a problem? When inquiring into the impact of intimate relationships on preventive behaviour it thus becomes necessary to reframe the unit of analysis. In preparation for our study we formulated the hypothesis that it is the intimate dyad, not the detached individual, who acts either preventively or non-preventively when faced with HIV risk, as detailed above.

Observing the system

How do you observe intimate systems empirically? How do you deal with the circular causality of a social phenomenon through which the phenomenon creates and transforms itself? Among the numerous decisions to be taken, four were particularly important:

1   To base the data collection on self-observations by the participants of intimate systems.
2   To focus these self-observations on a detailed reconstruction of the key event of the last sexual encounter experienced by the participants.
3   To use qualitative in-depth interviews for obtaining the information needed.
4   To explore dyadic intimate systems through in-depth interviews with just one of the partners. (This decision was made after we tested and rejected the alternative of interviewing both participants.)

The in-depth interviews covered three main topic areas:

1   A detailed reconstruction of the last heterosexual encounter, from petting and mutual masturbation to sexual intercourse.
2   A description of the intimate relationship in which the sexual encounter took place with a special focus on the communicative properties of the relationship.
3   An exploration of how the intimate partners actually dealt with the mundane problems of contraception, HIV, and condoms.

All three topic areas were explored by examining differences among the various sources and types of information gathered. Among these 'differences that make a difference' (an expression of Gregory Bateson; see Simon, 1988) the following were most important: the difference between perceptions on the cognitive level verses the information communicated on the social level; the difference between the participant and his/her intimate partner; the difference between erotic and non-erotic content; and time differences, such as before, during and after the encounter. The transcripts of the interviews were used as a basis for extracting both quantitative data, especially regarding the kind of HIV risk management performed, and qualitative information concerning the impact of communication on preventive choices.

Selecting and distinguishing

The basic systemic orientation predetermines not only the methods for gathering information, but also the methods for analysing the data. Although the analysis strives for the usual empirical ideal of the greatest possible generalisation, one finds that common scientific procedures of statistical analysis and abstraction often fail when they deal with research objects characterised by a high degree of interdependence and interaction. In such cases, the commonality which the objects of research – here the relational systems – have with systems of a similar type is superseded by their individuality and singularity (Eisenstadt *et al.*, 1995). The prevailing methods of scientific classification and generalisation demand that it be possible to reproduce each result. This presupposes an ontological reality independent of theory, a reality which is assumed to be linear and homogenous. In conceiving intimate relations as autopoietic social systems,[2] however, we make it clear that this reality:

1   is not static, but rather dynamic and procedural
2   is characterised less by continuity and fixed identity than by movement and heterogeneity, and
3   is not ontologically existent, but emerges out of interaction.

An intimate relationship only exists to the extent that it is observed and that it makes a difference to the observer (whether within or outside the couple). An analysis which takes this into account has to develop methods capable of perceiving the seemingly disorderly and confusing processes which keep reproducing themselves. It is exactly in this category of the chaotic and the confusing where we find intimate systems, not only from the perspective of the scientific observer, but also from the perspective of the partners in the couple.

Using the triangulation of quantitative and qualitative procedures, the analysis was conducted in two interrelated steps:

•   In the quantitative analysis, the observations of the interview transcripts were transformed into binary, categorical, or nominal data by a scientific observer, according to predefined criteria. These data are divided into two domains: (1) the main characteristics of the intimate system and (2) the concrete form of HIV risk management employed in the system.
•   The qualitative analysis identifies, with the help of hermeneutic procedures, individual processes in the construction of intimate communication and critical points for preventive action.

The typological categorisation and coding of the transcripts was done in different rating loops with at least two independent observers (of different gender), who were not identical with the interviewer. A congruence of observations was taken as a confirmation; a difference led to further analysis and a conclusive vote by the research team as a whole.

Results

Both the quantitative and the qualitative analyses show that the proposed model of four distinct modes of intimate communication – romantic, hedonistic, matrimonial, and prostitution-based – is well-suited to describing heterosexual intimate relations, thus offering a comprehensive typology for analysing the communicative dimension and social dynamics of intimate partnerships.

In the last sexual encounter, the least use of condoms was found in matrimonial and romantic intimate systems (the former slightly below, the latter slightly above 10 per cent of encounters). Higher levels of condom use were found in hedonistic systems (about 25 per cent). By far the most effective kind of preventive action was found in prostitution-based intimate systems, where in more than two out of three intimate situations a condom was used. Correspondingly, the lack of condom use was highest in matrimonial and romantic intimate systems (above 80 per cent), followed by hedonistic systems (*c.* 70 per cent), with prostitution-based systems at the low end with approximately 16 per cent. (See Table 10.1.)

The use of condoms, in spite of its being promoted by the public health system as the most effective prevention strategy, is but one form of HIV prevention in the internal workings of intimate partnerships. Besides condom use, there is a whole range of other forms of prevention which were catalogued and systematically ordered according to their presumed effectiveness. The result was a 5-point scale of HIV risk management behaviours. Coding the complex qualitative data into linear quantitative variables through standardised rating procedures it can be shown that specific HIV risk management behaviours are associated with the type of intimate system. Table 10.2 shows the particular forms of HIV risk

Table 10.1 Condom use by type of intimate system

	R	H	M	P	X	Total
Condom Used	3	10	4	26	3	46
	12.5%	26.3%	10.3%	83.9%	37.5%	32.9%
Condom Not Used	21	28	35	5	5	94
	87.5%	73.7%	89.7%	16.1%	62.5%	67.1%
Total n	24	38	39	31	8	140
	100.0%	100.0%	100.0%	100.0%	100.0%	100.0%

Note: Figures represent total number of couples in the respective category of intimate system, followed by the percentage of the total represented by the number. The total n is 140, as not all 161 interviews produced reliable information about condom use in the relationship.

management chosen by the intimate dyad during their last sexual encounter, distinguished by the four types of the intimate system.

If these data are condensed and transformed into a scale which includes only the most effective prevention strategy used by the system during the last encounter, the characteristic preventive profile of each intimate system become clear. The romantic type displays by far the least effective form of HIV risk management with two out of three intimate encounters including no preventive behaviour; whereas, the corresponding proportion lies considerably lower in matrimonial and hedonistic intimate systems (44 per cent and 34 per cent). Considering both Levels I and II as rather ineffective forms of prevention, H and M systems still lie below the 50 per cent line. Prostitution-based intimate systems stand out again as the type involving the least risk in terms of HIV, with less than 7 per cent of the sexual encounters taking place without protective behaviour. (See Table 10.3.)

The poor figures that lasting relationships (the M type) provide on Level V (10.3 per cent) must be seen in connection with the relatively high figures on Level IV (about 30 per cent). In marital relationships, strict monogamy represents the single most important form of risk management. Regarding the forms of HIV risk found on Levels V and IV as moderately effective, if they are actually performed, matrimonial intimate systems are equal with hedonistic ones (both about 40 per cent). Romantic intimate systems range again at the low end of the effectiveness scale; less than one-fifth of the last sexual encounters in this type used effective forms of HIV risk management. All the trends outlined here can be replicated also for the more generalised accounts of sexual behaviour beyond the last encounter.

As important as these figures are in terms of pointing out the association between the kind of HIV risk management observed and the type of intimate communication, this quantitative logic treats all intimate systems alike and thus tends to conceal the strong qualitative differences between them.

The omission of the condom may, for instance, be due entirely to different factors which are immediately connected to the basic operation of the intimate system. If the condom is indeed left out in a prostitution-based system (P), it is usually the result of negotiation initiated by the client. The prostitute only responds to a request not to use a condom if, for example, work is slow or if she has the impression that her competitors do it without. To cover the costs for the room, advertisements, food, etc., she may finally consent not to use a condom – even if this violates her professional norm – because she is in great need of money.

In marriages, which clearly belong to the M type, the necessity of preventive action only results if the relationship is no longer exclusive. As marriage is fundamentally based on exclusiveness, many couples find it difficult – even threatening – to face the fact that there is a third partner involved. As communication about extra-marital affairs is often considered to be impossible without endangering the relationship, preventive action can only be introduced with great difficulty.

Table 10.2 HIV risk management for the last sexual encounter categorised by level of effectiveness

Level of HIV Risk Management	Reported HIV prevention behaviours During the last sexual encounter	R	H	M	P	X
Level V	Use of condom	11.5%	25.0%	8.2%	68.4%	37.5%
	Avoidance of penetration	3.8%	10.0%	none	10.5%	12.5%
	Total	*15.3%*	*35.0%*	*8.2%*	*78.9%*	*50.0%*
Level IV	Strict monogamy	3.8%	5.0%	24.5%	none	none
	Total	*3.8%*	*5.0%*	*24.5%*	*none*	*none*
Level III	Sexual practices: abstention from anal intercourse and from penetration during menstruation	none	2.5%	none	none	none
	Limitation of the number of partners	11.5%	10.0%	12.2%	none	none
	Total	*11.5%*	*12.5%*	*12.2%*	*none*	*none*
Level II	HIV testing of one partner or both, but without observing the time period for seroconversion	none	2.5%	2.0%	none	12.5%
	Partner selection: avoiding partners in risk groups	3.8%	10.0%	2.0%	none	none
	Talking about HIV risks	3.8%	5.0%	6.1%	none	12.5%
	Total	*7.6%*	*17.5%*	*10.1%*	*none*	*25.0%*
Level I	Doing nothing; no preventive behaviour observable	61.5%	32.5%	34.7%	5.3%	37.5%
	No intimate interaction observed	7.7%	5.0%	20.4%	18.4%	none
	Total	*69.2%*	*37.5%*	*55.1%*	*23.7%*	*37.5%*

Note: Percentages indicate the proportion of couples in the category of intimate system who performed the behaviour during the last sexual encounter. As several couples undertook more than one preventive behaviour during the last encounter, percentages add up to more than 100% Level 1 is presumed to be the least effective category of HIV prevention behaviours, and Level V the most effective.

Table 10.3 The most effective form of HIV risk management employed during last
sexual encounter, catagorised by level of effectiveness

	R	H	M	P	Total
Level V	4	14	4	29	51
	16.7%	36.8%	10.3%	93.5%	38.6%
Level IV	1	1	12	—	14
	4.2%	2.6%	30.8%	—	10.6%
Level III	2	4	4	—	10
	8.3%	10.5%	10.3%	—	7.6%
Level II	1	6	2	—	9
	4.2%	15.8%	5.1%	—	6.8%
Level I	16	13	17	2	48
	66.7%	34.2%	43.6%	6.5%	36.4%
Total	24	38	39	31	132
	100.0%	100.0%	100.0%	100.0%	100.0%

Note: Figures represent the number of cases in each category with percentages indicating the proportion of couples in the category of intimate system who performed the behaviour during the last sexual encounter. Level 1 is presumed to be the least effective category of HIV prevention behaviours, and Level V the most effective. The residual category X has been excluded from the calculation of percentages. Due to rounding, the sum of percentages may be above or below 100%.

Intimate partners who are in love with each other (R type) may, on the other hand, find it easy to talk about AIDS in general. However, talking about AIDS does not often translate into preventive action for romantic intimate systems. Both partners feel so close, so intimate with each other. The partner is so much adored; he or she is seen as pure and perfect in the eyes of his/her partner, making protection against HIV unnecessary from the perspective of the system (compare 'risk factor love' in Dannecker, Chapter 11; Bochow, Chapter 12). Hedonistic relationships (H), on the other hand, are particularly confronted with the fragility of the (momentary) intimate interaction which is neither supported by nor embedded in a more comprehensive social relationship. To avoid ruining the fleeting erotic moment that both partners have been able to construct, they avoid a discussion of AIDS and condoms and hence act without any effective protection.

Discussion

Sexuality in general, and HIV preventive behaviour in particular, are characteristically marked by the social context of the intimate relationship and its dynamics. In the modern and post-modern societies of today, four basic types of intimate communication have evolved: romantic, hedonistic, matrimonial and prostitution-based intimate systems. These four types differ fundamentally in their communicative properties and constitute altogether different conditions for AIDS prevention.

An effective HIV risk management strategy for the intimate dyad is immediately connected to its communicative style. The level of intimate communication is key, determining whether intimate partners are able to talk about sexual topics; whether they can discuss such mundane problems as contraception, AIDS, and condoms; and whether or not they come to a common decision concerning preventive action. Without communication in advance to the sexual contact, no common preventive behaviour can evolve.

To describe intimate relations as autopoietic social systems of intimate communication sheds light on their basic mode of operation which bears important practical consequences for HIV prevention. Self-referencing systems which produce their own operations and react upon self-produced internal states are inherently difficult to influence from the outside. The concept of intimate social systems may thus help to promote a certain degree of realism regarding the possibilities of controlling intimate systems in their preventive behaviour through external intervention. Given the operational closure of the intimate system, every kind of preventive intervention can only take place in the environment of the system. However, the system defines the conditions under which it allows itself to be influenced from the outside. Preventive messages only have a chance of creating an impact if they are in line with the basic operations of the target system. To give an example: the condom forms an integral part of prostitution-based systems. Its lack of use is generally the result of negotiation on the part of the client. Training prostitutes in communication skills would help in rejecting such demands and at the same time increase the solidarity of the working women, a crucial element in prostitutes' yielding to lack of condom use, according to our interviews. (Compare Ahlemeyer, 1996.)

Being autopoietic in their operation, intimate systems are not easy to grasp. They are not trivial in the sense that they do not produce identical outputs from the same inputs (Geyer, 1992). Though somewhat constant in their basic operating mode of intimate communication, their structures are by no means unchangeable. In their operations, intimate systems can change their structure and even their mode of operation (Foerster, 1981).

The concept of intimate social systems may be more about understanding the complexity involved in the apparent trivial act of using a condom than about influencing condom use from outside, the latter being virtually impossible if one is striving for predictable and consistent results. Strengthening intimate systems in their ability to determine their own course must therefore be the foremost aim of HIV prevention policies. If the participants of intimate systems do not succeed in preventive modifications of their sexual behaviour, there is no one who can do it for them, neither the state nor the public health system.

There is, however, another implication of these findings. The analysis makes clear that preventive behaviour is complex, difficult to carry though, and dependent upon a whole range of situational and relational factors not completely under the control of the individual. Recognizing this challenging complexity may help to create support and understanding for those who have failed the task, who have not taken protective measures against an HIV infection and have thus contracted the virus. Such an impetus against stigmatisation and discrimination is in itself both important and practical.

Notes

1   For a more in-depth discussion of the methodology of the study see Ahlemeyer, 1995, 1997.
2   Intimate dyads are autopoietic systems; that is, systems which constantly produce and reproduce their constituative elements. Systems of this kind are immanently restless; they are exposed to a dynamic that is endogenously produced. An adequate point of reference for analysing them is thus not some presupposed balance or other static state, but rather the continuing reproduction of momentary events which are inherent to the systems. (See Geyer, 1992.)

References

Ahlemeyer, H. (1990) 'Intime Kommunikation und präventives Handeln: Über einige soziale Voraussetzungen der Primärprävention von Aids', in R. Rosenbrock and A. Salmen (eds), *Aids-Prävention*, Berlin: edition sigma: 181–7.
—— (1995) 'How to explore intimate systems?' in W. Heckmann (ed.) *AIDS in Europe*, Berlin: edition sigma.
—— (1996) *Prostitutive Intimkommunikation: Zur Mikrosoziologie hetero-sexueller Prostitution*, Stuttgart: Enke.
—— (1997) 'Observing observations empirically: Methodological innovations in applied sociocybernetics', *Kybernetics* 26(6/7): 641–60.
Bundeszentrale für gesundheitliche Aufklärung (BZgA) (1994) *AIDS im öffentlichen Bewußtsein der Bundesrepublik*, Cologne: BZgA.
Cupach, W. and Metts, S. (1989) 'Sexuality and communication in close relationships', in K. McKinney and S. Sprecher (eds), *Human Sexuality. The Societal and Interpersonal Context*, Norwood, N.J.: Ablex: 139–61.
Eisenstadt, P., Hurth, D. and Stiehl, H. (1995) *Wie Neues entsteht: Die Wissenschaft des Komplexen und Fraktalen*, Reinbek: Rowohlt.
Foerster, H. (1981) 'On self-organizing systems and their environment', in H. von Foerster, *Observing Systems*, Seaside, Calif.: Intersystems: 1–23.
Gerhards, J. and Schmidt, B. (1992) *Intime Kommunikation. Eine empirische Studie der Annäherung und Hindernisse für 'safer sex'*, Baden-Baden: Nomos.
Geyer, F. (1992) 'Autopoiesis and Social Systems', *International Journal of General Systems* 21: 175–83.
Heckmann, W. and Koch, M. (eds) (1994) *Sexualverhalten in Zeiten von Aids*, Berlin: edition sigma.
Koch, M. G. (1987) *AIDS: vom Molekül zur Pandemie*, Heidelberg: Spektrum.
Küppers, G. (1994) 'Experimentelle Steuerung: Kalkulierbare Eingriffe in die Selbstorganisation', in Beratergruppe Neuwaldegg (ed.), *Planung als Experiemt*, Vienna: Service: 13–34.
Luhmann, N. (1984a) *Liebe als Passion. zur Codierung von Intimität*, Frankfurt/Main: Suhrkamp.
—— (1984b) *Soziale Systeme. Grundriß einer allgemeinen Theorie*, Frankfurt/Main: Suhrkamp.
McKinney, K. and Sprecher, S. (eds) (1991) *Sexuality in Close Relationships,* Hillsdale: Lawrence Erlbaum.
Simon, F. (1988) *Unterschiede, die Unterschiede machen. Klinische Epistemologie: Grundlagen einer systemischen Psychiatrie und Psychosomatik*, Berlin: Springer.
Weeks, J. (1986) *Sexuality*, Chichester: Ellis Horwood.
Willke, H. (1987) 'Strategien der Intervention in autonome Systeme', in D. Baecker *et al.* (eds) *Theorie als Passion*, Frankfurt/Main: Suhrkamp: 333–62.

11   The 'risk factor love'

Martin Dannecker

Introduction

The promotion of HIV prevention among homosexual men is certainly one of the most successful health campaigns to be instituted over the last several decades. However, in spite of the impressive success of interventions targeted to this population, prevention efforts have not been as effective as was hoped. This is not seen so much in the annual rate of new infections in Germany, which has stabilised (see Marcus, Chapter 3), but rather in the relatively constant level of risk contacts in certain contexts of homosexual life. Prevention efforts for homosexual men were clearly most successful precisely where they were predicted to fail; namely, in relation to casual sexual contacts. HIV prevention has enjoyed less success, however, in the context of steady relationships between men. On the basis of the empirical data gathered to date, one could characterise the development of a committed relationship between men as a situation which promotes risk behaviour, thereby making the individuals involved more susceptible to an HIV infection. Ironically, love has turned out to be a risk factor (Dannecker, 1990; Davies *et al.* 1993; Schiltz and Adam, 1995; Bochow, 1997).

Casual contacts and love relationships

One can speak of two different forms of sexuality when comparing ongoing relationships with casual encounters. The difference between the two only becomes apparent when we avoid equating safer sex with condom use. The data which I gathered in 1987 (Dannecker, 1990) already indicated that homosexual men tend to rely more on avoiding higher risk practices (or, at least, practices which are viewed by the individual as higher risk) than on condom use as a means to prevent infection. This was at a time when the sexual repertoire of homosexual men had been severely limited as a result of AIDS. Whereas, before AIDS a large proportion of homosexual men practised a relatively broad spectrum of behaviours (mutual masturbation, receptive and/or insertive oral and anal intercourse); AIDS resulted in the limiting of the sexual repertoire to mostly mutual masturbation and oral-genital contact. This means that anal-genital sex with or without a condom is now far less commonly practised by homosexual men than before

AIDS made its debut. Of course, anal sex does continue to occur, but this behaviour no longer constitutes an essential feature of homosexual relations as it did for a large proportion of men before the epidemic.

This form of prevention by avoidance, if you will, characterised by limiting the type of practices performed, is found predominantly within the context of casual sexual contacts (for example, in parks, public restrooms, highway rest stops, backroom bars, and in saunas). In contrast, this form of prevention is found less often in ongoing relationships. Condom use also plays a far less important role in anal sex between steady partners than between men having sex outside of such relationships (Dannecker, 1990; Bochow, 1997).

Although the higher exposure to HIV risk within steady relationships among homosexuals has been known for some time, it is only recently that this dynamic has become the subject of prevention activities. Up to this point, the focus of prevention has been on casual homosexual encounters and the inherent infection risks in such situations. The general public has labelled such casual sex between men as 'promiscuity', which has been viewed by some to be abnormal. This view is based on the simple observation that homosexual men on the average have a higher number of sexual partners than their heterosexual counterparts. This 'promiscuity' has been described as being an important factor in the transmission of HIV, with the crude descriptor 'large number of partners' being equated with a high risk for infection. This 'promiscuity', with the associated anonymous and fleeting contacts, was said to be the motor driving the epidemic. This emphasis on homosexual 'promiscuity' turned out to have an important influence on how HIV risk was constituted in general, and on the risk perception of homosexual men, in particular. This resulted in a belief that steady partnerships present a relatively lower level of risk. Of course, this belief was never formulated as such. Rather, the talk was of a 'different risk rationale' in unprotected sexual contacts with 'steady partners' versus contacts with anonymous partners. Implicitly, the notion was that this 'different risk rationale' or 'different risk management strategy' was easier to apply than the risk management employed during 'promiscuous' sex. In this way the stereotype was supported that anonymous, fleeting encounters are risky; whereas, 'steady partnerships' are safe.

Even the AIDS service organisations in Germany, the AIDS-Hilfen, promoted this dichotomising of HIV risk through their prevention campaigns. For a long time, the immense AIDS education program for homosexual German men concentrated exclusively on topics which were directly connected to casual sex. This can be seen not only in the images of homosexuality found on the 'safer sex posters', but also in the forced sexualised language in the various brochures. The exclusive focus of prevention was a form of sexuality which had been 'freed' from any connection to love or romance. However, in spite of careful attempts to present exclusively the sexual aspects of such encounters in the various prevention media, the message was clear that even this form of sex needed to be kept an eye on. In retrospect, one can view this obvious sexualisation of homosexual encounters as being a form of denial of the restrictions which AIDS had placed on sexuality. However, it is precisely in supporting this denial by means of concentrating exclusively on the sexual aspects of safer sex that HIV prevention within anonymous encounters achieved its success. HIV prevention for homosexual men targeted the 'pure' sexuality which takes place outside of relationships. This 'pure' sexuality is performed for its own sake, unencumbered by the constraints imposed by the various dimensions of an ongoing relationship. Above all, this form of sexuality rejects the limits imposed by the demands of love. It is this sexuality freed of love, as lived by certain segments of the homosexual subculture, which has been the exclusive domain of the safer sex campaigns of the AIDS service organisations. The result has been the ignoring of the other side of homosexual sex; that is, the sexuality which is lived within relationships. More precisely, HIV prevention for homosexual men has isolated the two sides of men's sexuality from one another. Prevention efforts have thus artificially separated from each other the intertwined infection risks associated with both casual encounters and sex within a relationship.

The problem of love

As we know, based on several years of research on homosexuality, gay men tend toward being in a relationship, and gay men in a relationship tend toward promiscuity (Dannecker and Reiche, 1974; Dannecker, 1990). This reality complicates HIV risk management tremendously, because all strategies need to take into account both having sex within and outside of an ongoing relationship. Prevention for anonymous encounters appears to be relatively easy and straight forward: anyone who is HIV-negative, or who believes himself to be negative, is risking an infection if he has sex with a new partner whose HIV status he does not know. But because one cannot be sure of the partner's status, HIV prevention has propagated the practical rule of thumb that one should generally avoid having anal intercourse or use a condom. The fact that most men cannot always keep to this rule does not detract from its practicality in anonymous encounters.

Avoiding anal sex or using a condom with new partners is very useful because we have no reason to trust someone whom we do not know. Of course, one who believes himself to be negative could ask a new partner about his HIV status directly. But could he trust the answer? Probably not. We would be more likely to believe the answer to this question if it came from a person whom we love. We tend to trust those whom we love, even when we know that this trust is illusory. Just like everyone else, homosexual men idealise those with whom they share a love relationship. One of the consequences of this idealisation is that a great deal of trust is placed in the person. Another consequence is the inner conviction that the one whom I love would do nothing to hurt me or to make me sick. Without such a conviction a relationship based on love is not possible. We are describing here an illusion which is necessary for the couple. This illusion and the trust which it entails applies also to the risk for HIV infection which one or the other partner brings into the relationship. Therefore, it is deceptive to think that someone in a love relationship will be able to obtain reliable knowledge about his partner's previous or concurrent sexual contacts. And the assumption that each individual can be in charge of his own preventive behaviour in every situation amounts to a delusion of grandeur. (See Ahlemeyer, Chapter 10.) Even in the so-called open relationships, one cannot assume that the partners are able to talk about everything which is associated with HIV risk, including previous and current sexual contacts. This is true in spite of the appearance that such relation-ships have forsaken the typical expectations of love and fidelity, explicitly negotiating the types of contacts permissible outside of the couple.

Indeed, as compared to heterosexual relationships, one finds in homosexual relationships a great deal more doubt regarding promises of fidelity and all the fantasies and desires which are characteristic of the ideal of romantic love. This doubt is also likely to be more conscious among homosexuals than among heterosexuals. One finds in many homosexual relationships explicit knowledge of sexual contacts which one or the other partner has outside of the couple; and this is often accompanied by an agreement, which may have more the quality of a concession, that such contacts should be permitted under certain circumstances (Dannecker, 1990). This, however, does not mean that the ideal of romantic love has been eliminated from homosexual relationships; this ideal continues to have an influence, albeit inconspicuous. Even though homosexual relationships are not as a rule monogamous, the idea of fidelity is far stronger and more prevalent than all appearance would suggest. The majority of homosexual men share the general cultural attitude toward infidelity, in spite of their sexual practices (Dannecker, 1990). This attitude dictates that sexual infidelity places love in danger. Because sexual infidelity is also experienced by homosexual men in this way, they, too, will at least to some extent hide or deny aspects of their sexual contacts outside of the couple, including potential HIV risks.

So we find that the ideal of romantic love is also a problem for homosexuals when it comes to following through with behaviour prescribed by the logic of prevention. The difficulty arises precisely in that moment when two people fall in love because 'being in love' is a special psychosomatic state which relativises all external reality as well as all precepts from the surrounding culture. Being in love literally makes one anti-social. It is for this reason that in the phase of being in love all prior relationships and sexual encounters lose their meaning. No matter who or what came before, the one who is happily in love sees everything in the past as meaningless; this applies to his own history as well as to that of his partner. It is, therefore, hardly possible when one is in love to maintain a realistic perspective on one's own sexual history and that of his partner as demanded by the rationale of prevention.

In my experience counselling homosexual men, the relationship to one's own sexual history and to that of one's partner is generally restricted in the early phases of being in love. In the beginning of the relationship, any reticence regarding prior sexual contacts or potential HIV risk results in the avoidance of higher risk sexual practices or in the use of condoms. Over time, however, the representation of the loved one changes: he goes from being the 'Unknown' to being the 'Trusted One'. Through this transformation the previous preventive behaviours become less consistent; this takes place first in one's thoughts and later in reality. According to the findings of Michael Bochow (1997) 54 per cent of homosexual men in relationships lasting one to six months use a condom for every act of anal intercourse. The longer the relationship, the lower the frequency of using a condom regularly. In relationships which have lasted for more than two years, the proportion of men regularly using a condom for anal intercourse is only one-fourth, with 56 per cent not using a condom at all when having sex with their steady partner. (See also Bochow, Chapter 12.)

The increasing lack of preventive behaviour in relationships over time does not, however, necessarily mean that the risk for HIV is increasing proportionally. It may very well be the case that the probability that a couple is jointly tested for HIV increases over time, as well. In any case, the reduction in preventive behaviour which accompanies a relationship is based on a feeling of safety which is rooted in trust. This feeling of safety found in relationships is, however, largely due to a mystification. This mystification is closely connected with love, the latter blinding us, enchanting us, beguiling us – because we want to be blinded, enchanted, and beguiled. And we are not only subjected to the power of this mystification when we are in love with someone. This mystification also exerts its influence when we view love from the outside, for example, in the role as researcher. In the latter situation we tend to emphasise the lucid, tame, beautiful – and in the case of AIDS – safe side of love, denying or at least minimising its dark, conflict-ridden and ugly side. This tendency can be seen in HIV prevention research which for many years assumed that unprotected anal-genital sex in the relationships of homosexual men was performed according to 'the golden rule of prevention', without critically examining whether this was, in fact, the case.

In recent years there has been mounting evidence that 'the golden rule' is not followed in steady partnerships. Accordingly, a large proportion of new infections are likely to be the result of higher risk sexual contacts in relationships which are defined by the men involved as steady partnerships or which are, at least, of the kind in which the possibility of love is fantasised and desired. In other words, where sex is accompanied by love, the probability of risk contacts and therefore of HIV infection is higher than in sexual encounters which are characterised by a pure sexual interest, that is, by the view of the partner as a sexual object as opposed to an object of love (Dannecker, 1990; Kleiber and Velten, 1993; Davies *et al.*, 1993; Bochow, 1997).

The couple as its own entity

In answer to the question why HIV prevention is less reliable among couples than within the context of casual sex we can say that, as discussed thus far, there is the essential problem of bringing together prevention with love. The latter would mean depicting the loved one as a potential disease carrier. The second reason is that there have simply been too few prevention messages directed specifically to the homosexual couple. Up to this point, HIV prevention has been largely focused on the psychology of the individual with the result that prevention messages have been targeted to individual men. One has assumed that this strategy would strengthen couples in their intention to protect themselves. A couple is, however, not only more than the some of its parts, but also something other than the two individuals involved. A couple is a third entity which is relatively independent of the two partners. The couple, as its own entity, confronts the two individuals in the relationship with its own dynamic and with specific challenges to act. Thus being in a couple can modify behavioural intentions of the individual partners, including the intention to protect oneself or one's partner from HIV.

In psychoanalytic terms, the couple as a third entity is seen as the unconscious of the couple. From a systems theory perspective the couple can be described as a social system. Heinrich Ahlemeyer (Ahlemeyer and Puls, 1994; Ahlemeyer, 1996; see also Ahlemeyer, Chapter 10) and his research group have applied the systemic concept of Niklas Luhmann to HIV prevention research. Ahlemeyer and his colleagues were able to support empirically their hypothesis that not only characteristics of individuals in a couple, but also factors related to the couple as an intimate system are essential elements in preventive behaviour. The findings of Ahlemeyer *et al.* suggest that an intimate system is capable of modifying the behavioural intentions of the individuals in the couple. The various types of intimate systems appear to have differing capacities to influence the preventive intentions of the individual partners. In particular, a steady partnership is most likely to affect the individual's ability to act on his/her own initiative. This means that in the context of a love relationship one can act in ways which are contrary to his/her previous intentions.

In light of these findings, one can surmise that there is a stronger influence on a homosexual man's preventive intentions in the context of a love relationship (steady partnership) than in casual sexual contacts with other men. This may be the case because preventive measures within the steady partnership are tied to fears and fantasies which see prevention as a latent threat to the relationship. Evidently, the main influence on HIV prevention in couples is not the wish to avoid infection, but rather, the conscious or unconscious threat posed to the couple's relationship. Even the most well-informed couple (given that the couple's relationship is relatively intact) is interested both in avoiding HIV infection and in maintaining the relationship. Apparently the physical distance imposed by HIV prevention is experienced as being more limiting in a love relationship than in casual contacts. In the latter, the distance imposed by preventive behaviour affects the sexual experience but it does not threaten the bonds of love.

Toward the future: breaking the taboo

There are, however, not only differences in risk exposure between sexual contacts in relationships versus those with other partners. We also find differences among couples regarding risk behaviour. In order to understand these differences it would be necessary to conduct research on the steady partnerships of homosexuals. This would allow for identifying various criteria related to risk-taking as well as differentiating between the various types of partnerships and the various cycles within a partnership. This differentiated view may allow, for example, for an enhanced ability to address problems in preventive behaviour related to crises within the life cycle of the couple. On the basis of such empirical data it would be possible to target prevention efforts to specific aspects of love relationships among homosexuals. However, this issue continues to remain practically taboo. Paradoxically, it is the widespread belief that homosexual men are incapable of ongoing relationships based on love which is standing in the way of seeing how important love really is and taking the necessary steps toward more effective HIV prevention.

References

Ahlemeyer, H. (1996) *Prostituitive Intimkommunikation. Zur Mikrosoziologie heterosexueller Prostitution. Beiträge zur Sexualforschung* vol. 74, Stuttgart: Enke.

Ahlemeyer, H. and Puls, W. (1994) 'Typen intimer Kommunikation in der heterosexuellen Allgemeinbevölkerung', in W. Heckmann and M. A. Koch (eds), *Sexualverhalten in Zeiten von Aids*, Berlin: Enke.

Bochow, M. (1997) *Schwule Männer und AIDS. Eine Befragung im Auftrag der Bundeszentrale für gesundheitliche Aufklärung,* Berlin: Deutsche AIDS-Hilfe.

Dannecker, M. (1990) *Homosexuelle Männer und Aids. Eine sexualwissenschaftliche Studie zu Sexualverhalten und Lebensstil,* Stuttgart, Berlin and Cologne: Verlag W. Kohlhammer.

Dannecker, M. and Reiche, R. (1974) *Der gewöhnliche Homosexuelle. Eine soziologische Untersuchung über männliche Homosexuelle in der Bundesrepublik,* Frankfurt/ Main: S. Fischer Verlag.

Davies, P. M., Hickson, F. C. I., Weatherburn, P. and Hunt, A. (1993) *Sex, Gay Men and AIDS,* London: Falmer Press.

Kleiber, D. and Velten, D. (1993) *Prostitutionskunden. Eine Untersuchung über soziale und psychologische Charakteristika von Besuchern weiblicher Prostituierter in Zeiten von AIDS,* Baden-Baden: Nomos Verlagsgesellschaft.

Schiltz, M. A. and Adam, P. (1995) *Les homosexuels face au SIDA: Enquêtes 1993 sur les modes de vie et la gestion du risque VIH,* Paris: CAMS, CERMES.

Part IV
Responding to specific target groups

12 The response of gay German men to HIV

The national gay press surveys, 1987–96

Michael Bochow

Introduction

The Deutsche AIDS-Hilfe (DAH), the National German AIDS Organisation, was founded in September 1983 in West Berlin. Following the first prevention campaigns in 1984 and 1985, the need was identified to investigate to what degree the information materials had affected the knowledge and behaviour of gay men in Germany. To this end, Gerd Paul, then board member of the DAH, contacted the author in 1986 to discuss the design of a study. It was decided in the summer of 1987 to implement a questionnaire based on an instrument used by Michael Pollack in his survey of gay French men conducted in 1985 and 1986 through the magazine *Gai Pied*, the leading gay publication at the time in France. (See Pollak, 1988, Schiltz, 1998.) The initial survey conducted in West Germany through the gay German press yielded such useful information that a second wave was commissioned for 1988. Starting in 1991 the Federal Centre for Health Education (*Bundeszentrale für gesundheitliche Aufklärung, BZgA*) took over the financing of this ongoing study of gay men, a national sample being collected at regular intervals through the gay press. This article provides an overview of the results of the waves conducted in the 1990s with a particular emphasis on the most recent data collected in 1996. The next scheduled collection of data is the end of 1999.

The sample

In July 1996, for the fifth time since 1987, a 4-page questionnaire was circulated by the most important gay magazines in Germany. The survey asked gay men about their sexual behaviour under the impact of AIDS. This was a replication of the version of the survey that had been carried out in November 1991 and December 1993.

A total of 3,048 men participated (514 or 17 per cent from eastern Germany, including East Berlin and 2,534 or 83 per cent from western Germany, including West Berlin). Forty-five per cent of the participants lived in the four German cities with a population of one million or more (Berlin, Hamburg, Munich, and Cologne). Twenty-one per cent of the participants lived in cities and towns with less than 100,000 residents. The highest level of education was distributed as follows (percentages represent the associated diploma or its equivalent): 11 per cent primary school diploma, 24 per cent 10th grade diploma, and 65 per cent pre-university diploma (39 per cent have a university degree, 17 per cent are college students). These percentages indicate that men having ended their education at primary school and those living in smaller cities and towns are under-represented in the sample; however, there are enough participants from both of these groups to be included in the statistical analysis. The mean age of the participants was 34.9 (median: 33).

Method

It is still not possible to conduct a representative study of men who have sex with men, even for those men who identify as gay. In spite of substantial progress in Western and Central European societies, homosexual behaviour continues to be a largely hidden phenomenon, with gay men being the focus of discrimination and marginalisation. (See Bochow 1997a.)

Given this limitation, measuring the behaviours and attitudes of gay German men in light of HIV has been particularly problematic. A nationwide survey conducted through the gay press has proven to be the best solution for obtaining valid and reliable data. Replication of the study at regular intervals since 1987, along with making use of interregional and international comparison of results, has ensured the quality of the data and a balanced interpretation of the findings.

The surveys conducted in 1987 and 1988 in West Germany along with those conducted in 1991, 1993, and 1996 in united Germany show a large degree of stability in the socio-demographic structure of the sample. The samples do, however, under-represent gay men over 44 years old and men with little contact to the gay community (not only men in rural areas but also men in the cities who have little contact to community structures). The tendencies found in the surveys can, nevertheless, serve as indicators for trends over time among homosexually-active men in Germany, as the men who are most active socially and sexually (the men who could be considered 'trend-setters') are over-represented. As in France (see Schiltz 1993; Schiltz and Adam 1995) the questionnaires were distributed through the gay press, as this is the most efficient method to obtain a large sample from all regions in the country. Interestingly, the results obtained reflect those found using the method of conducting standardised interviews as reported in Australia and the UK (Kippax *et al.* 1993; Davies *et al.* 1993).

Type of partnership and HIV risk

Anal intercourse and type of partnership

All national studies of gay men in Germany since 1971 show that about four-fifths of the respondents practice anal intercourse at least 'sometimes,' whether as the receptive partner, as the insertive partner, or playing both roles. (See

Dannecker and Reiche 1974; Bochow 1988; Dannecker 1990; Bochow 1994.) In 1996, 81 per cent of the West Germans surveyed and 82 per cent of the East Germans had at least occasional anal-genital contact. The percentage of men who did not practice anal intercourse in the last twelve months is highly dependent on the relationship status of the subjects. Twenty-seven per cent of the men without a steady partner at the time of the study reported no anal-genital contact; whereas, only 15 per cent of the men in a closed (monogamous) relationship and 10 per cent of the men in open (non-monogamous) relationships did not have anal intercourse over the last year.

Fifty-four per cent of the men practised both receptive and insertive anal inter-course. Ten per cent had exclusively receptive and 17 per cent exclusively insertive anal sex. The flexibility of the sexual repertoire is also dependent on the partnership status of the subjects. Forty-five per cent of the men who were not in a steady relationship had both receptive and insertive contact; whereas, 58 per cent of the subjects in (for the most part) monogamous partnerships and 65 per cent of those in non-monogamous relationships assumed both roles during anal intercourse. The proportion of men who have exclusively insertive or receptive sex is not dependent on relationship status.

Not only the incidence of sexual contact, but also its frequency, appears to be associated with the type of relationship. In looking at all sexual practices as a whole, we find that 42 per cent of the men in steady partnerships had sexual contact several times a week; whereas, only 14 per cent of the men not in a primary relationship had sex this often. Thirty-five per cent of the men in steady partnerships had sex several times a month with their primary partner or with other partners; only 24 per cent of the men without a steady partner had sexual contact with this frequency. This indicates that three fourths (77 per cent) of the men in primary relationships had sex several times a month or more often; whereas, only 38 per cent of the men without steady partners reported this frequency of sexual contact.

In analysing anal-genital contacts there appear to be even greater differences based on partner status. Thirty-seven per cent of the men in steady relationships (representing 20 per cent of the total sample) had anal-genital contact several times a month or several times a week. Fifteen per cent of the men not in a steady rela-tionship (representing 12 per cent of the total sample) had anal-genital contact with this frequency. When all responses are tabulated we find that 27 per cent of the sample had frequent anal-genital contact.[1] This percentage is comparable to that found in the wave of the national survey administered in 1993 (see Bochow 1994).

Frequency of risk behaviour and type of partnership

Only twenty-one men (0.7 per cent of the sample) did not respond to the question regarding unprotected anal intercourse with partners whose HIV status they did not know. The number of subjects is somewhat higher (thirty-eight men; 1.2 per cent of the sample) who did not answer the follow-up question regarding which partner was involved and at what frequency the unprotected sex occurred.

Seventy-seven per cent of the West Germans and 74 per cent of the East Germans reported not having had unprotected anal intercourse in the last twelve months with a partner whose HIV status they did not know. Ninety-six per cent of both the West and East German samples did not have unprotected anal intercourse with a partner whose HIV status was different than their own. A total of 76.4 per cent of the West Germans and 72.4 per cent of the East Germans did not have either of these two forms of risk contact in the last year. As compared to 1993, this represents a stable pattern of safer sex behaviour among the West Germans (no risk contacts in 1993: 75.9 per cent) and a slight increase in safer sex behaviour among the East Germans (no risk contacts in 1993: 70.3 per cent). When looking at safer sex compliance trends since 1987, the following picture emerges:

The results of the studies conducted in 1991 and 1993, as well as the results of other research in Germany (Dannecker, 1990) and in Western Europe (for example, Bochow *et al.,* 1994; Davies *et al.,* 1993; Schiltz, 1993; Schiltz and Adam, 1995), show that anal intercourse – including unprotected anal intercourse – occurs predominantly in steady partnerships (Bochow, 1994).[2]

The results of the German survey in 1996 strongly support the above observation. Twelve per cent of all subjects reported unprotected anal-genital contact with a steady partner whose HIV status was unknown to them. This risk was taken by 5.5 per cent of the total sample once a month or more often as shown in Table 12.2. Nine per cent of the men surveyed had unprotected anal intercourse with non-steady partners whose status was unknown to them (excluding anonymous encounters). This risk was taken by 0.7 per cent of the men (twenty subjects) once a month or more often. Eleven per cent of the men had anonymous unprotected anal sex with partners of unknown status. This situation was reported by 0.6 per cent of the sample (twenty subjects) as having occurred once a month or more often.

· These data show that a significant percentage of the men (23 per cent) have risk contacts with partners whose serostatus is unknown to them. The percentages

Table 12.1 Selected results from the German gay press survey

Year of survey	n	Median age contact	Percentage without risk	Percentage tested for HIV	Percent HIV-positive
Western Germany					
1987	924	30	61	52	10.8
1988	1122	30	63	57	12.0
1991	2630	30	69	63	11.2
1993	2393	30	76	69	10.3
1996	2534	33	76	73	10.8
Eastern Germany					
1991	655	30	59	39	5.3
1993	475	30	70	55	6.5
1996	514	32	72	63	8.6

Table 12.2 Anal intercourse without a condom, serostatus of sex partner unknown, survey year: 1996

Anal intercourse without a condom, serostatus of partner unknown	n	%
Total yes	693	22.7
Total no	2,334	76.6
No response	21	0.7
Total	3,048	100.0
With a steady partner		
1–4 times total	141	4.6
5–10 times total	57	1.9
Once/week-once/month	168	5.5
Not applicable	2,682	87.9
Total	3,048	100.0
With casual partners		
1–4 times total	217	7.1
5–10 times total	42	1.4
Once/week-once/month	20	0.7
Not applicable	2,731	90.8
Total	3,048	100.0
With anonymous partners		
1–4 times	282	9.2
5–10 times	26	0.9
Once/week-once/month	19	0.6
Not applicable	2,721	89.2
Total	3,048	100.0

Note: Subjects were asked to report on sexual activity within 12 months prior to the survey.

also clearly indicate that, for the large majority of men who risk HIV infection (four-fifths), taking risk with non-steady partners is a sporadic occurrence (one to four times a year). This observation makes clear how meaningless it is to describe such sporadic events as 'relapse into unsafe behaviour'. For the men who report one to four unsafe sexual contacts with casual or anonymous partners, most of their sexual behaviour actually consists of protected anal intercourse, mutual masturbation, or oral sex. The sporadic risk contacts are, therefore, exceptions which do not represent a 'relapse' or return into a phase of increased unprotected behaviour.

Even in steady partnerships, risk-taking in terms of HIV infection is rather the exception than the rule. The highest frequency of risk contacts is, however, found among this group. Of the men in steady partnerships who engaged in risk-taking: 46 per cent had risk contacts once a month or more often, 16 per cent five to ten times, and only 38 per cent had sporadic risk contacts (that is, one to four times in the last twelve months).

As noted above, 23 per cent of the respondents (26 per cent of the East Germans and 22 per cent of the West Germans) had at least one incident of unprotected anal-genital contact with a partner of unknown serostatus. A much smaller percentage of men (3.2 per cent) reported unprotected anal intercourse with partners whose serostatus was different from their own (3.5 per cent of the East Germans, 3.1 per cent of the West Germans). These highest risk contacts also take place at a higher frequency within the context of the steady relationship. However, the differences related to partner status are not as great for serodiscordant encounters as for sex with partners of unknown status.

Condom use as a regular part of sexual practice

Four-fifths of the men (78 per cent) who had anal sex in the last year with non-steady partners reported that they always use condoms during anal intercourse. It can be stated that these men have integrated condom use as a regular part of their sexual practice. A further 15 per cent of these men reported that they use condoms frequently. These respondents can be described as having adopted condom use as part of their sexual practice, but condom use each time is not a given. Eighty-five per cent of the men in the sample reported using a condom during their last act of anal intercourse with a non-steady partner. There are no differences regarding frequency of condom use based on role played during intercourse (receptive, insertive, or both).

Within steady partnerships there is a considerably smaller portion of men who regularly use condoms. Only one-third (35 per cent) of the men who had anal sex with their steady partner always use a condom. Forty-six per cent report never using condoms. Whether or not a condom is regularly used is dependent on the length of the steady relationship. Fifty-four per cent of the men with relationships of one to six months always use a condom when having anal intercourse (29 per cent never). Where the relationship has lasted seven to twelve months, the percentage of men regularly using condoms falls to 44 per cent, with the percentage of men never using condoms rising to 38 per cent. In relationships of over two years, regular condom use drops to one-fourth, and those never using condoms is at 56 per cent. There is a similar trend concerning the use of condoms during the most recent act of anal intercourse with a steady partner.

Summary

The findings presented to this point concerning partnership and risk lead to the following conclusions: it is not the often discussed promiscuity of gay men in the 1980s – that is their 'fast lane' lifestyle of having multiple partners – which results in a high incidence of risk, but rather the psychosexual dynamic of the steady partnerships of which they are a part. The incidence of risk within steady partnerships is considerably higher than that within casual encounters. The affective dynamic of more intimate and committed sexual relationships excludes the distant, calculated risk management which can take place during casual sex.

The different dynamic of such intimate relationships, as opposed to more casual contacts, has been discussed in Germany by Martin Dannecker (see Chapter 11) and in Sweden by Benny Henriksson (1995) using the term 'risk factor love', based on qualitative research which they conducted. Particularly Dannecker has emphasized that permanent relationships often are accompanied by the fantasy of unity and permanence, regardless of whether the relationship proves to be a lasting one in reality. The feeling of love which develops – or which is at least fantasised – in steady relationships can nullify the more careful management of risk which one finds during casual sex. For gay men with permanent relationships, the condom may symbolise not only the presence of AIDS; it can also be seen as an unbearable barrier to intimacy with the partner. Both aspects can lead the partners to refrain from using the condom. Seen in this light, the desire for trust and intimacy – like the desire to escape the dictates of the prevention 'commandments' – plays a much greater role in sexual interactions with steady relationships. The feeling of being kept apart by the condom is much easier to bear in sexual interactions outside of permanent relationships than in love relationships. The feeling of being in love temporarily neutralises the impulses that exercise control. Therefore, the strong affective colouring of sexual interaction in a love relationship often leads to patterns of behaviour that are different from those seen in casual sex. Casual sex interactions are much more open to conscious control and individual risk management.

This, of course, does not mean that casual sex contacts are completely unproblematic as far as risk-taking behaviour is concerned. Rewarding casual sexual interactions may contain the *promesse de bonheur* of a steady relationship. Permanent relationships and casual contacts are not separated by some insurmountable barrier. Fantasy is invariably a factor which can influence action. Even a fantasised intimacy can lead to risk-taking behaviour during a casual sexual contact. The sexual fantasies that develop out of psychological and physical needs have to be taken into consideration in the analysis of sexual interactions, as does the influence of subconscious processes that are beyond conscious controls. Consequently, even in the case of casual sex, unprotected anal-genital contacts can mean that the distancing from the partner, which may be symbolised by the use of a condom, is being avoided. (See summary in Bochow, 1995.)

HIV-testing and risk-minimising strategies

One of the questions in the 1996 survey focused on the motivation to have oneself tested for HIV. The possible responses included 'I would like to stop using a condom when having sex with my steady partner'. The result: 27 per cent per cent of all respondents had themselves tested for HIV to find out if they had the same serostatus as their partner so they could stop using condoms in their relationship. But for men in steady relationships, this percentage is even higher, namely 38 per cent. This high percentage is evidence for the large number of men who experience condom use as being a disruptive factor in the intimate relationship with their steady partner. In fact, not only men in steady partnerships report that condoms disrupt their sexual relations. Questions were included in the survey regarding attitudes toward condom use. For the sample as a whole, only one third of the men (34 per cent) who had anal sex feel that condoms 'do not disrupt' or 'hardly disrupt' their sexual relations; whereas, one fifth (19 per cent) feel very restricted and almost one half (46 per cent) report a moderate level of disruption.

Social class and HIV risk

Surveys based on a self-administered questionnaire have by their very nature a built-in middle class bias. The surveys in 1991, 1993, and 1996 produced a series of convenience samples in which men with lower educational and occupational status, and working class men were clearly under-represented in relation to the importance of these groups in terms of the social structure of the overall population. Even so, we may note that the absolute numbers of returned questionnaires are sufficient in themselves to insure that under-represented subgroups of the overall gay population were available for meaningful statistical analysis.

Three class-groups were constituted using data on secondary education and occupational status:

1   Lower class: men with a secondary school diploma and an unskilled occupation.
2   Lower middle class: men with skilled vocational training or other comparable vocational qualifications.
3   Middle class: men with senior high school and technical college or university certificates (including students who have not yet finished their studies).

Upper class men, to the small extent that they may have participated in the survey, are included with the middle class men. Table 12.3 shows the sample composition by class for the surveys of 1993 and 1996.

Class-specific differences in the life styles of gay men in Germany

To analyse the extent to which the survey participants were leading an openly gay life, an 'openness index' was constructed based on questions such as: whether the

Table 12.3 Sample composition by class

Region and year of survey	Lower class		Lower middle class		Middle class		Total	
	n	*%*	*n*	*%*	*n*	*%*	*n*	*%*
Western Germany								
1993	175	7	859	36	1,359	57	2,393	100
1996	259	10	974	38	1,301	51	2,534	100
Eastern Germany								
1993	26	6	236	50	213	45	475	100
1996	26	5	261	51	227	44	514	100

mother, father or siblings of the respondent knew about his homosexuality and whether they accepted it; and to what degree the respondent's friends and co-workers were informed. It became apparent that lower class gays in both parts of Germany live in a substantially more covert manner than their middle class counterparts. Less than half of German lower class men live in a relatively open fashion and for the most part enjoy acceptance in their social environment; in contrast, two-thirds of German middle class men live openly as gay men and feel accepted by their social environment. There is almost no difference between networks of friends in the lower and middle class regarding their composition, be it exclusively of gay men, of heterosexuals of both sexes, or of an equal mixture of both. Nevertheless, it becomes evident that a greater proportion of lower class gays (one-tenth) lead socially isolated lives; whereas, only about 4 per cent of middle class gay men stated that they have no close friends.

In 1993 and 1996 a smaller percentage of lower class gays in both western and eastern Germany lived in a steady relationship than middle class respondents (roughly 45 per cent versus 55 per cent). On the other hand, in the twelve month period before the survey, the lower class group did not have more sexual partners than the middle class one. (Overall, for both eastern and western Germans from the lower and the middle classes, 16 per cent had one partner, 27 per cent had two to five partners, 16 per cent had six to ten partners, 30 per cent had 11 to 50 partners, and 9 per cent had more than 50 in the past year. Three per cent had no partners.) This suggests that at least the self-identified gay men from the lower class do not have substantially more anonymous sex than their middle class counterparts; however, when we consider the frequency of sexual contacts, class differences become more apparent. Less than half of German lower class men have frequent (several times a month or more) male-to-male contact, whereas two-thirds of the middle class respondents have frequent homosexual contact. We note here that explanations for less frequent sexual activity among lower class gay men should also be understood as being related to class-specific factors. A higher proportion of lower class gay men live in small towns and cities; a lower proportion of them live in steady relationships. Both these factors reduce their chances of sexual contacts. The western German group of lower class respondents is large enough to allow for further differentiation with respect to places of residence. Even a more stringent analysis still reveals that in cities of more than one million inhabitants, lower class men report less frequent sexual contact than their middle class counterparts. Middle class men without a steady relationship report higher rates of sexual contact than their lower class counterparts. A higher proportion of lower class men stated that in the twelve months prior to the survey they had no anal-genital contact. This again is related to the fact that, at the time of the survey, fewer lower class respondents were living in a steady relationship than middle class respondents.

To summarise: regarding a general exposure to HIV risk (excluding potential preventive behaviour), we may say that lower class men in Germany are exposed to fewer risks than middle class men with regard both to the frequency of sexual contacts and the frequency of anal-genital sex.

Class-specific differences in risk behaviour and risk strategies

Seventy-six per cent of western German and 72 per cent of eastern German respondents (1993: western Germans 76 per cent; eastern Germans 70 per cent) stated in 1996 that in the twelve months prior to the survey they had no unprotected anal-genital contact with persons a) whose test status they were unaware of, or b) who had a discordant test status from themselves.

Analysis of the 1996 western German sub-sample revealed clear class-specific differences. Sixty-nine per cent of lower class men, 75 per cent of lower middle class men, and 79 per cent of middle class men stated that they had not had sexual contact involving risk. For the eastern German sub-sample the respective figures are: 46 per cent, 71 per cent, 77 per cent. These differences are statistically significant at the 0.05 level.

Among men of lower socio-economic status we find not only more subjects who risked HIV infection, but also a greater percentage of men with a high frequency of risk contacts (over fifteen risk contacts in the last twelve months). Table 12.4 shows this class-related difference as reflected in unprotected anal intercourse with partners whose HIV status is not known, regardless of type of partnership. This comparison was possible because information concerning the frequency of the risk contact for all types of partners (steady, non-steady, and anonymous) was collected using the same method.

Class-specific differences in HIV-prevalence

There are marked differences between the three socio-economic groups regarding the percentage of HIV-positive men in the survey of 1996. Among the western Germans 20 per cent of the lower class men are HIV-positive, as opposed to 13 per cent of the lower middle class men and 7 per cent of the middle class men (among the 73 per cent of the western Germans who were tested).

Table 12.4 Socio-economic status and frequency of risk contacts with partners of unknown serostatus (western Germany, including West Berlin)

Socio-economic status	Number of risk contacts					No response	Total
	None	1–5	6–15	16–35	60–180		
Lower class n = 259	69.5	13.5	7.3	1.9	5.8	1.9	10.2
Lower middle class n = 974	76.0	12.5	5.6	1.1	3.5	1.2	38.4
Middle class n = 1,301	79.5	11.1	3.9	0.8	3.7	1.0	51.3
%	77.1	11.9	4.9	1.1	3.8	1.2	100
n	1,954	301	125	27	97	30	2,534

Note: all figures in per cent unless otherwise stated.

The percentage of HIV-positive men among the tested western German respondents were in 1993 as follows: 17 per cent for the lower class; 13 per cent for the lower middle class, and 8 per cent for the middle class. Thus, the prevalence of men with HIV infection or with AIDS is twice as high among respondents of the lower class than among middle class men. Figures for the eastern German sub-samples revealed no clear class-specific differences in either survey. This reflects the more egalitarian social structure still found in eastern Germany. In addition, it should be noted that the overall rates of HIV infection are much lower in eastern as compared to western Germany. (See Marcus, Chapter 3; Herrn, Chapter 13.)

In order to examine the effects of age, the western German samples from 1993 and 1996 were divided into three groups: a) 16–29 years old; b) 30–44 years old; and c) over 44 years old (most of the subjects in this age group are 45–65 years old). In the 1993 wave there is no evidence of class-related influences among the over 44 group. Strong class-related differences regarding infection rate are apparent, however, in the age groups 16–29 and 30–44. A chi-square analysis reveals a significant association for both of these age groups between socio-economic status and being HIV-positive ($p < 0.05$). (See Bochow, 1997a.) Within the 1996 data this association is significant for all three age groups ($p < 0.05$). Table 12.5 shows the class-related differences for all age groups of the western German men who had been tested.

Implications for primary prevention work

Ulrich Biechele is the author of the first German study on the preventive behaviour of men in the lower classes. His work is based on qualitative interviews, providing valuable complementary information to the quantitative data presented here. Biechele sees experienced gay men as being gatekeepers to the gay community. These are the men who, for example, do not merely go to the park in order to pick someone up and satisfy their sexual needs but who also feel a sense of responsibility toward other men in the gay community (Biechele, 1996). Biechele suggests more emphasis be placed on outreach work in primary prevention for lower class homosexual men. This work would be an adjunct to the use of print media and television advertising.

In light of Biechele's work and the findings of the Gay Press Survey, we can

Table 12.5 Percentage of HIV positive western Germans by age and socio-economic status

Socio-economic Status	Age 16–29	30–44	45 +	Total (1996)	Total (1993)
Lower class	11.9	17.3	30.4	19.6	17.1
Lower middle class	9.4	15.3	15.1	13.3	13.1
Middle class	3.1	9.0	7.9	7.0	7.9
n	573	1,002	272	1,847	1,654

draw some conclusions to guide future prevention work for this neglected population. The greater distance displayed by lower class gay men to the 'gay scene', the lower likelihood of being identified as gay (see Bochow, 1997a; Dowsett, 1996), and their specific communication and interaction styles all require a range of specially designed informational and counselling options. Broad appeals through the mass media or the distribution of printed material can only have a very limited impact on this population. What is called for are special forms of prevention activities based on outreach models. Information, counselling, and support agencies are needed that are adapted to the needs of this specific subgroup. Just what organisational structures and profiles such agencies should take remains to be seen. However, whatever form they may have, it will be vital for them to secure the engagement of activists who either have the same class background as the men they are trying to reach or who have developed a particular social proximity to them.

Drug use and risk behaviour

For the first time since the start of the Gay Press Survey, questions were asked in 1996 regarding the use of drugs such as cannabis, Ecstasy, LSD, heroin, cocaine and crack. Among the men surveyed there are very few consumers of heroin and crack. Cannabis is used 'rather often' by 7 per cent of the subjects, 'occasionally' by 19 per cent. One or more of the four so-called 'party drugs' (Ecstasy, speed, LSD and cocaine) are used 'rather often' by 2.5 per cent of the men and 'occasionally' by 8.5 per cent. A considerably higher percentage of the men who use cannabis and party drugs report risk contacts (approximately a third) as compared to the other subjects (approximately one-fifth). However, more frequent use of these substances does not necessarily mean higher risk behaviour, as two thirds of the men using party drugs and over two thirds of those using cannabis did not risk HIV infection during sex.

For this reason, prevention campaigns should avoid promoting a 'rule of abstinence' as part of the safer sex canon. It may be more effective to emphasize the potential loss of control during drug use. In order to reach the target groups this message needs to be adapted to the sensibility and lifestyles of the men using the drugs. AIDS prevention needs to recognise that the how and why of drug using in the larger cities is strongly connected to an adventure-seeking way-of-life which values particular communication norms and emotional styles. Within the context of HIV prevention it is particularly important for the techno subculture that communication skills be promoted which are adapted to a pleasure-seeking lifestyle. This focus is necessary to ensure that prevention messages are readily received within this group.

Conclusion

In this article an attempt was made to identify the various contexts of higher HIV risk found among gay German men based on the national survey conducted through the gay press from 1991–6. These contexts are characterised by such varied social-psychological dimensions as poverty, a lack of cultural capital, hedonism and the use of drugs, the ideal of romantic love, and the psychodynamics of gay relationships. It would be foolhardy to construct a risk model based on a factor analysis of these various dimensions. Such a model would produce some such constellation as working-class gay men in a steady relationship who smoke hash together will indubitably become infected with HIV and die. Risk does not necessarily occur in the presence of the characteristics described in this analysis. HIV prevention – not only for gay men, but for other groups, as well – can only be successful when conducted in the context of social and health policy measures which support the strength of the individual to act independently and in solidarity with others. Responsibility for oneself and risk-conscious behaviour thrive in societies with a high level of social cohesion and in the presence of communal solidarity. Protecting oneself demands self-confidence and self-esteem, both of which are based on being valued from important others in society. Successful HIV prevention therefore requires far more than well-thought-out strategies for primary prevention developed according to current models for public health practice. The success of HIV prevention in Germany is to be understood as the result of a social welfare system which ensures that a majority of the population enjoy at least a minimal level of participation in the wealth of the society.

One must also understand that health is not a goal for people, but rather 'only' a necessary pre-condition for one's goals in life to be realised. For example, sexual interactions do not, as a rule, have hygiene as their focus. The sanitary logic of HIV prevention can stand in contradiction to the internal logic of sexual interactions.

The basic structural problem with AIDS prevention, on both a programmatic and personal level, is the contradiction between the desire for intimacy, manifesting itself in a need for love and sexual expression, and the demand for a certain degree of autonomy, which is the prerequisite for successful risk management practices. In order to deal effectively with these opposing poles there is no golden rule in sight, any more than there are eternal truths to be revealed in defining the myriad psychosocial co-factors associated with HIV risk behaviour.

The task for prevention work is to uncover and interpret the different 'grammatical structures' of communication in various scenes and ways of life. This grammar has to be taken from the contexts in which it is practised. Although social science can describe the nature of risk management, including areas of deficiency, this cannot take the burden away from AIDS prevention organisations to develop and test appropriate concepts for the various subcultures for which they have a responsibility.

Notes

1   The figures 20 per cent and 12 per cent cannot be simply added because 5 per cent of all respondents had frequent anal sex with both their steady partner and other partners.
2   Regarding the structure and meaning of anal sex among gay men see the pertinent analysis of de Zwart, van Kerkhof and Sandfort (1998).

References

Biechele, U. (1996) *Schwule Männer aus der Unterschicht. Sexuelle Identität und HIV-Prävention*, Berlin: Deutsche AIDS-Hilfe.

Bochow, M. (1988) *AIDS: Wie leben schwule Männer heute*, Berlin: Deutsche AIDS-Hilfe.

—— (1989) *AIDS und Schwule. Individuelle Strategien und kollektive Bewältigung*, Berlin: Deutsche AIDS-Hilfe.

—— (1993) *Die Reaktionen homosexueller Männer auf AIDS in Ost- und Westdeutschland*, Berlin: Deutsche AIDS-Hilfe.

—— (1994) *Schwuler Sex und die Bedrohung durch AIDS – Reaktionen homosexueller Männer in Ost- und Westdeutschland*, Berlin: Deutsche AIDS-Hilfe.

—— (1995) 'Data deserts and poverty of interpretation. Notes on deficiencies in prevention-oriented research, taking gay men as an example', in D. Friedrich and W. Heckmann (eds), *AIDS in Europe – The Behavioral Aspect* vol. 4: *Determinants of Behavior Change*, Berlin: edition sigma: 249–57.

—— (1997a) *Informationsstand und präventive Vorkehrungen im Hinblick auf AIDS bei homosexuellen Männern der Unterschicht*, Berlin: Deutsche AIDS-Hilfe.

—— (1997b) *Schwule Männer und AIDS*, Berlin: Deutsche AIDS-Hilfe.

Bochow, M., Chiarotti, F., Davies, P., Dubois-Arber, F., Dür, W., *et al.* (1994) 'Sexual behaviour of gay and bisexual men in eight European countries', *AIDS Care* 6(5): 533–49.

Dannecker, M. (1990) *Homosexuelle Männer und AIDS. Eine sexualwissenschaftliche Studie zu Sexualverhalten und Lebensstil*, Stuttgart/Berlin/Köln: Verlag W. Kohlhammer.

Dannecker, M. and Reiche, R. (1974) *Der gewöhnliche Homosexuelle. Eine soziologische Untersuchung über männliche Homosexuelle in der Bundesrepublik*. Frankfurt/Main: S. Fischer Verlag.

Davies, P., Hickson, F. C. I., Weatherburn, P. and Hunt, A. J. (1993) *Sex, Gay Men and AIDS*, London, New York/Philadelphia: Falmer Press.

Dowsett, G. (1996) *Practicing Desire. Homosexual Sex in the Era of AIDS*, Stanford, Calif.: Stanford University Press.

Henriksson, B. (1995) *Risk Factor Love: Homosexuality, Sexual Interaction and HIV Prevention*, Gothenburg: University of Göteborg.

Kippax, S., Connell, R. W., Dowsett, G. W. and Crawford, J. (1993) *Sustaining Safe Sex: Gay Communities Respond to AIDS*, London: Falmer Press.

Pollak, M. (1988) *Les homosexuels et le SIDA. Sociologie d'une épidémie,* Paris: Editions A. M. Métailié.

Schiltz, M. A. (1993) *Les homosexuels masculins face au SIDA. Enquêtes 1991–1992.* Paris: CAMS, CNRS.

—— (1998) *Les homosexuels face au SIDA: Enquête 1995, Regards sur une décennie d'enquêtes*, Paris: CAMS, CERMES, CNRS.

Schiltz, M. A. and Adam, P. (1995) *Les homosexuels face au SIDA: Enquête 1993 sur les modes de vie et la gestion du risque VIH*. Paris: CAMS, CERMES.

Zwart, de, O., van Kerhof, M. P. N. and Sandfort, T. G. M. (1998) 'Anal sex and gay men: The challenge of HIV and beyond', in M. T. Wright, B. R. S. Rosser and O. de Zwart (eds), *New International Directions in HIV Prevention for Gay and Bisexual mMen*, New York: Haworth Press: 89–102.

13 Western-style prevention for eastern gay men?

AIDS prevention in the former East Germany

Rainer Herrn

Introduction: the difference between East and West

With the fall of the Berlin Wall the separation of Germany came to an end, and the situation concerning AIDS in the eastern part of the country changed completely. On the one hand there were fears that the welcomed political change could lead to an uncontrollable spread of HIV in the former East Germany. On the other hand, there was hope among activists in the East that AIDS prevention strategies – particularly those for gay men – would be improved, setting up a system comparable to that in West Germany. Up to that point in time, the Wall had functioned epidemiologically as a protective barrier, the amount of contact with epicentres in the West being severely restricted. AIDS prevention targeted to gay men had also been generally neglected because of the ignorance of East German state institutions, including the health system, regarding social minorities and their potential for self-help. Table 13.1 summarises the differences between the national strategies of East and West Germany regarding the prevention of HIV for gay men.

In East Germany gay men were not regarded as a special target population. Their need for specific information and education in the form of lifestyle-oriented print media was neglected. In addition, there was a lack of financial and institutional support for AIDS service organisations. Finally, the existing gay networks were disregarded when prevention messages were designed and disseminated.

In contrast, West Germany decided in the mid-1980s for a liberal prevention strategy, following a brief but highly charged national debate concerning the use of isolation and containment for infected persons. (See Frankenberg and Hanebeck, Chapter 4.) This resulted in prevention for gay men becoming a priority for state funding, with AIDS service organisations (the AIDS-Hilfen) being established at the local, regional and national levels. By the early 1990s, the AIDS Service Organisations (ASOs) had developed the concept of *structural prevention* to serve as the theoretical underpinning for their work. (See Etgeton, Chapter 7.) The preventive work of the ASOs focused on supporting diverse gay lifestyles and developing context-specific interventions and media.

Another important distinction between East and West Germany regards the

Table 13.1 Comparison of the HIV prevention strategies for gay men in East and West Germany before 1989

	East Germany	West Germany
Target group	Homosexuals and heterosexuals viewed as being equally at risk.	Homosexuals defined as a group in need of special attention. AIDS Service Organisations funded at all government levels, with gays identified as a primary target group
Prevention message	Emphasis on monogamy in relationships. Promiscuity defined categorically as a riskisexual practice (even with a condom).	Emphasis on safer sex strategies promoting anal sex with condoms and oral sex without exchange of semen. No recommendations to discourage anal intercourse as a practice or the frequency of sexual contacts
Medical vs. social paradigm	Emphasis on medical interventions to contain and control HIV (mass screenings, partner tracing, testing of gay men). Neglect of social and political dimensions of AIDS, including the needs of special populations.	Emphasis on social and political dimensions of HIV. Testing with counselling. Test as a decision of the individual. Differentiated prevention messages and mediums for different populations and settings.

Note: The categories in the table are adapted from Rosenbrock, R. (1994) 'Strategie und Politik für wirksame AIDS-Prävention', *AIDS-FORSCHUNG* 9(2). 9 85–90.

content of prevention messages and the role of medicine in controlling the spread of the disease. Whereas a control and containment strategy was present in East Germany, including both mass screening and the discouragement of sexual activity, the western approach promoted sex-positive messages about avoiding specific risks. Further, testing was viewed sceptically in the West, given the potential negative psychological consequences of a positive test and the lack of effective treatment. Emphasis in West Germany was placed on informing individuals, particularly in specific target groups, of the risk of infection and providing them with the support to make their own decision regarding testing.

In summary, the East German prevention strategy was closely patterned on the traditional approach to fighting sexually transmitted diseases. This is in contrast to the West German prevention strategy, where group-specific educational interventions were aimed at strengthening individuals' skills for managing infection risks. This difference in approach has been summarised by Rosenbrock *et al.* (1999) as the 'old' versus the 'new' public health. (see also Rosenbrock *et al.*, Chapter 20.)

Because of the fear of a rapid increase of HIV infections in East Germany, the country's first ASO (*AIDS-Hilfe DDR*) was founded in 1990. This organisation was later subsumed into the structures of the Deutsche AIDS-Hilfe (the National German AIDS Organisation), becoming the Department for Eastern Germany. Additionally the Federal Ministry for Health in Bonn commissioned the special AIDS programme 'East' from 1992–4 in order to establish the West German AIDS prevention strategy in the East German public health system. Over ten years later, there are no longer any special programmes promoting HIV prevention in the former East Germany, neither through governmental nor non-governmental bodies. Currently, there are approximately fifteen local ASOs in eastern Germany which are members of the Deutsche AIDS-Hilfe. The dreaded spread of the AIDS epidemic to the eastern part of the country did not occur.

In the years 1987 to 1989, the years just before the Wall fell, the incidence of HIV in East Germany was thirty cases in the entire country, while in the same period there were about 6,000 positive HIV tests reported in West Germany. The comparatively low incidence of HIV in the eastern region of the country has remained consistent, even following unification. (See Table 13.2).

After unification, we see an increase of new HIV cases in the eastern part of the country and a continued gradual decrease in the western region. An important goal of HIV prevention must be the maintenance of a low prevalence of HIV in the East. Regardless of these differing prevalence levels, gay men comprise the most affected group in all parts of the country. Maintaining the low level of infection in the East will depend largely on the ability of gay men to protect themselves, which implies a need for special prevention measures for gay men. Interestingly, recent quantitative research shows a slightly higher distribution of risk practices regarding HIV infection amongst eastern gay men as compared to their western counterparts. Repeated cross-sectional studies indicate, however, that the differences between East and West regarding risk-taking behaviour are declining (Bochow, 1997). The author of these studies, Michael Bochow, concluded from his results.

A concept for the primary prevention in the new Länder [the former East Germany] which takes their specific situation into account has not been presented by the Deutsche AIDS-Hilfe or the local AIDS-Hilfen [ASOs] in East Germany until now. It remains an urgent desideratum and should be developed and discussed by the Deutsche AIDS-Hilfe.

(Bochow, 1993: 37)

Table 13.2 Epidemiological data: HIV in Germany, new cases reported by year and region

	1993	*1994*	*1995*	*1996*	*1997*	*1998*
Former West Germany	2,318 cases 95.9%	2,164 cases 92.7%	2,104 cases 92.4%	1,723 cases 90.4%	1,891 cases 90.2%	1,566 cases 92.8%
Former East Germany	98 cases 4.1%	170 cases 7.3%	173 cases 7.6%	183 cases 9.6%	205 cases 9.8%	122 cases 7.2%
Total cases	2,416	2,334	2,277	1,906	2,096	1,688

Source: National AIDS Surveillance Centre, Robert Koch Institute, Berlin.
Notes: The figures for the years 1997 and 1998 are not final due to the delay in reporting and the percentage values are for the national total for both parts of the country.

Instead of developing a strategy specific to the needs of the eastern part of the country, the prevention model that had been used successfully in the West was simply applied to the East, disregarding situational and cultural differences.

For western models of prevention to be successful in the East, there would need to be strong similarities between gay men in both parts of the country. One needs to assume that gay men in the eastern part of the country have quickly adapted to the political upheaval by assuming western gay norms regarding lifestyle, communication, commercial enterprise and subcultural institutions. What one finds, however, are persistent differences between the gay subcultures east and west. This raises several questions: was application of the western prevention strategy successful in spite of the unique characteristics of the target population? Are the current prevention strategies suitable? What is the level of acceptance of prevention messages by gay men in the East? And finally, to which extent did gay men translate their preventive knowledge into preventive behaviour?

Sample and method

To answer these questions the Federal Ministry for Health commissioned a research project to investigate the structures of communication, the forms of socialising, and the current lifestyles of gay men in the eastern part of the country in order to have the necessary information to propose improvements in AIDS prevention for that region. By using qualitative research methods based in grounded theory (see Reisbeck *et al.*, 1993; Strauss *et al.*, 1996) the AIDS preventive behaviour of eastern German gay men can be understood in terms of the situational context and biographical experience of the individual subjects. This theoretical perspective allows for interpretation of the data under two aspects: the history of the individual and the structures of local gay life. A summary of the study's findings will be presented here. (For the full report of the data see Herrn, 1999.)

The sample was drawn from eight cities in eastern Germany to reflect the diversity of population size, geographical location, distance to large metropolitan gay centres, and extent of gay infrastructure which one finds in that part of the country. Within these cities a total of forty-one partially structured interviews were conducted. In larger cities eight to nine interviews were realised; in mid-size and small cities, three to six interviews. Only in Hoyerswerda was it impossible to find more than one interview partner, given the fear gay men have there of coming forward and openly discussing their situation. Both men well-connected to local gay institutions and those living less openly were interviewed. All subjects were recruited through contact persons which the author had known through gay networks in the former East Germany. These persons were well-informed about the diverse local gay subcultures. The author proceeded to build the purposive sample by specifying to the contact person the characteristics he was seeking in an interview partner (for example, amount of contact to the gay scene, age, level of education, time of coming out, social network and relationship status) and subjects were referred by the contact person. The sample was recruited in such a way as to reflect a diversity of East German men. All but five interviews took place face-to-face in the subject's home; the locations of the five other interviews were different because two of the men were married and one was living with his parents. The interviews, ranging from 80 to 190 minutes, were recorded on cassette and partially transcribed for analysis. The subjects had an age range of 21–71 years old. Three-quarters of the men (thirty subjects) identified themselves as gay (some only after the Wall fell); however, all subjects had sex with men. Ten identified themselvdes either as 'homosexual' (the usual self-label in East Germany) as 'queer', 'other', or rejected self-definition. Two subjects were HIV-positive; for one of these men the interview was the first time he had spoken with someone about his serostatus. Most (thirty-five) of these men had their coming out under the former East German political system. Additionally, fifty interviews were conducted with informants from the local gay communities to provide detailed descriptions of subcultural structures and norms. (For a more detailed description of the sample and method of the study see Herrn, 1999.)

Eight interviews were selected for this chapter to describe problems encountered by the men in the sample in appropriating the differing prevention messages before and after the Wall fell, that is, the different messages in East versus West Germany. Presented here are selected quotations from the interviews with accompanying interpretation (based on the data of the study as a whole). The excerpts were chosen to provide examples of themes encountered during the course of the investigation. This material does not pretend to describe comprehensively the problems of gay men in eastern Germany regarding HIV prevention nor does it propose a more general typology of reactions of gay men concerning AIDS in that part of the country. However, the selections indicate important issues which warrant more thorough investigation.

Themes from the interviews

One of the interviewed men was a nurse born in 1927. He has had sexual contact with boys and men since his youth in the Nazi period. He was strongly identified with the ideology of the East German state. He was sentenced to prison for several years for having sexual contact with patients. Later, he married and had several children, not identifying as gay until after the Wall fell. This subject commented on his personal prevention strategy by saying 'I've basically always gone barefoot,' meaning he does not use condoms for anal intercourse, even with new partners. This man, living in a village from his birth until now, is attempting to salvage the past by maintaining his habitual behaviour and attitudes from the period before the Wall fell. He has neither changed his philosophical stance (comparing Nazi Germany to East Germany) nor sought out new experiences. For example, he has only been to the Black Forest (in the West) once to visit his brother since the Wall fell. His attachment to the way things were in East Germany includes suppressing the demands of prevention promoted since unification. Although he says 'I'm into giving blow jobs', and 'I mostly get fucked',

– practices comprising HIV risk – he stated 'If I were totally honest I'd say I've never been with one single man who's used a condom – not once in my whole time with men'. The lack of safer sex compliance directly supports his denial of infection risk. In addition, this interview partner preferred state measures of control (for example, mass screenings) over personal responsibility. This is a reflection of elements of the East German AIDS prevention strategy working at the individual level.

Another man, born in 1958, a university lecturer in Marxism at a college in Thuringia, and an active member of the East German gay movement, commented 'After being tested we can do it without condoms as long as we trust each other'. This is a typical example of an internalisation of the central prevention message in East Germany 'Faithfulness is the best protection'. This man reported that he clearly prefers long-term partnerships. He avoids sexual contacts outside of a relationship, having difficulty accepting sexual contacts between his partner and other men, as well. In his last relationship, he believed his partner was having 'unsafe' sex with others; but in spite of this suspicion, he was not able to talk with his partner about it nor to insist on condom use when they had sex. Instead, he had himself re-tested as a response to his fear of infection. This interviewee said that he also wanted to practice 'faithfulness as the best protection' in his next relationship, going together with his partner to be tested.

Another man in the study, born in 1963, was living in a large city in Saxony. He was originally trained in sales but was working as a decorator at the time of the interview. This subject commented 'The motivation to protect myself didn't come until I somehow felt affected by the disease'. This statement is illustrative of two common experiences in East Germany; namely, the lack of contact with HIV (due to the low sero-prevalence) and the resultant lack of behaviour change, even after the unification of the country. This subject said:

> And after the Wall fell it took a while for people to feel like it had anything to do with them. And of course everyone, even me, has thought that it couldn't happen to him. I know all the people I sleep with and I know who they've been with. That was always the East German mentality because nothing could come in from the outside.

Only after this subject fell in love with an HIV-positive man from the West did he become more conscious of his behaviour. Direct experience with the disease following unification seems to have been most important in terms of men adopting preventive behaviour. This interview makes clear that this type of behaviour is not restricted to rural areas, but that it is also found among gay men in the larger cities who have experience in the gay subculture.

Another gay man, born in 1966, lives today in a small village where he works as a cook in a pub. He is very self-confident and reported sexual contacts only with 'people I know' and anal sex 'only with friends I've known a long time'. His commentary reveals a very widespread and important prevention strategy in the East: 'Of course I would use it [a condom] with strangers, but with strangers it just doesn't get that far'. Many gay men in the eastern part of the country rely on their relative isolation from the epicentres of the virus. They still think in terms of the East German 'epidemiological island' which existed when the Wall was still intact. The men assume that sex with those whom they 'know' is not dangerous, as opposed to sex with strangers, particularly with those from 'outside'. The real strangers for this man are the West Germans whose behaviour is difficult for him to figure out. He said he would 'never' let himself become sexual with West German men because 'those people are a little reckless [. . .] [but] act as if they're as pure as snow'.

Another man, born in 1971, was the 'baby' of the family in a city in a regional capital in the southern part of East Germany. He learned his trade as a butcher and then studied to be a geriatric nurse's aide. Today he feels himself part of the alternative scene, remarking 'I've started always doing it without [a condom]'. This man later emigrated to a larger city with a gay subculture where he for the first time met men who protected themselves from HIV infection. His comment is typical for the behaviour of many, showing the considerable deficits in condom use in the East. Today he says,

> If I would change, have sex on the side, then I'd make sure to do it [have sex with a condom]. Before [in the early 1990s in his home town] that wasn't possible; I never thought about it and I trusted the people. That probably wasn't the right thing.

In concordance with the national AIDS prevention strategy in East Germany, it was recommended that gay men take the HIV test. Test-taking and reliance on external recommendations is evident to this day in the personal prevention strategies of many man. The willingness to be tested in these cases shows a trust in the actions of the government and a willingness to delegate one's own responsibility to the health system and the state. Indeed, some even believe the HIV test to be a kind of treatment for the disease. The proportion of gay men from eastern Germany who have been tested for HIV has risen continually over the last several years. In 1996, a national study reported 63.2 per cent of eastern German gay men reported having been tested as compared to 72.9 per cent of their western German counterparts (Bochow, 1997). Considering, however, the much lower prevalence of HIV in eastern Germany this proportion of men tested is surprisingly high, suggesting that the motivation for testing described here is playing an important role.

In short, interviews with gay men who came out in East Germany suggest that the post-unification prevention measures do not replace prior prevention strategies, but rather modify them, leading in many cases to contradictory preventive behaviours which have yet to be addressed by prevention campaigns. Interviews with men who had their coming out after unification indicate that gay men who had not been exposed to East German prevention measures have significantly fewer problems in adopting the safer sex strategy promoted after 1989.

Not all of the difficulties which gay men have in adopting an effective individual prevention strategy have their roots in factors specific to the East German experience. Many gay men in both the East and the West fail to translate their knowledge into preventive behaviour because such a change involves the sensitive and complex area of sexuality, which is not simply subject to rational decision-making concerning risk exposure. (See Dannecker, Chapter 11; Ahlemeyer, Chapter 10; Bochow, Chapter 12.)

For example, one of the interviewed men (born in 1965) lives a hidden life. He is rejected by his family because of his homosexuality and does not want people in the supermarket where he works to know about his sexual preference, so he has a 'girl friend' act a cover. He said: 'I can't always trust myself'. He describes himself as someone who will not dare to approach men he is attracted to. So he developed a strategy as a youth of going to sexual meeting places like public restrooms and other public sex areas where men would come up to him. He now has the impression of not being attractive enough any more, because men do not come up to him as often. Therefore, he does not frequent the places of public sex as much. Concerning his sexual preferences he said 'I'm totally anally fixated, because I always met guys who liked doing "that" with me and I liked having "that" done to me'. But nowadays when he does have sex he said,

> Now I want it, now I need it, and then I'm (whistle). Whenever I'm in a situation and there's no condom around and the guy is really nice physically then you think in the back of your head this isn't someone who's promiscuous.

This underlines the difficulties of consistent follow-through even in the presence of adequate knowledge.

Information deficiencies are evident in an interview with a man born in 1967. He was earlier part of the national socialist youth group co-ordinating structure and today works in banking. He comes from a privileged East German family from a large city in the north. He is also HIV-positive. Regarding sexual risk he said 'What are the limits?' Like many other gay men, this man expresses his sexual needs on the weekends in Berlin – more precisely in East Berlin – allowing him to keep his sexual life separate from his place of residence and his work. Although he is well-informed about AIDS and infection risks he has difficulties in defining the boundary between 'safe' and 'unsafe' sex practices, particularly since he has found out he is HIV-positive. Although recent studies indicate that gay men in both the eastern and western parts of the country are well informed about HIV risk (Bochow, 1997), this quotation makes clear that there continues to be a need for education and information. Outreach-oriented methods may be most appropriate to address areas of uncertainty regarding the level of safety of specific practices. He says,

> I think the most important thing is that you talk about it. [. . .] Then the issue is out there and in people's head, because you just throw the [prevention] material in the corner. Most important is being able to ask questions about it.

This man expresses a preference for prevention in the form of interpersonal communication which one finds often in the former East Germany. He also identifies the urgent need for gay men collectively to deal with the disease, something which did not take place in East Germany.

Gay life in eastern Germany

The research project was not only devoted to identifying individual deficiencies in HIV prevention but also to analysing the specific conditions in which prevention for gay men takes place. The second part of the study contains detailed descriptions of gay life in selected locations, discussing the modification of AIDS prevention required to address the special situation in the East. Such modifications have to do with specific content, locations, and methods for prevention. For this purpose a more precise description of the various forms of gay life is fundamental.

In order to explore the differences between the various cities and towns, the characteristics of gay life in different places were compared. Even towns of equal size show differences in subcultural norms and structures which can be traced to East German influences. The explanation for the difference between the gay subcultures in East and West has two variations: There is a time lag in the East or the subculture in the East resembles that in rural areas in the West. Both interpretations are pejorative and only detract from seeing the differences in development regarding gay life due to forty years of division.

Analogous to the presentation of the individual interviews above, the sketches of the local communities are summarised here by characteristic quotations from gay men who live there.

The information gathered in Leipzig, after Berlin the second largest city in the East and considered the clandestine gay capital in East Germany (population 545,307 in 1988, decreasing to 478,200 in 1996 due to emigration from the city) indicates that 'exclusively gay pubs have no tradition in this town'. This is a likely reason why the predicted expansion of the western gay pub and bar culture did not occur in eastern cities. Gay men in the East seem to prefer the traditional so-called 'mixed' (gay and heterosexual) pubs and bars over gay establishments, at least in their own home towns. This explanation for preference varies from place to place. In Leipzig as elsewhere in East Germany several pubs with a largely gay clientele were closed in a short period of time. Gay pubs were undesirable. Because of this East German gay men did not have experience with a gay pub culture. In addition, creating gay ghettos is rejected by some men socialised in East Germany. One subject from Leipzig said concerning gay pubs,

> It is an homogenous, closed-off system of people [. . .] who hardly communicate with one another. I got bored of that pretty quickly. The mixed [gay and heterosexual] meeting places which already existed in great number in Leipzig before the Wall fell are much nicer because they're livelier and it's easier to get in conversations with people.

What this means concretely for HIV prevention is that there are no suitable locations in most communities for distributing explicit gay-oriented printed material and for interpersonal methods of intervention, because of the limited freedom for talking about such issues as compared with the West. The men interviewed named the following reasons for the lack of exclusively gay pubs and bars in the East:[1]

- The migration of men interested in the gay subculture to cities in western Germany.
- The satisfying of sexual needs away from one's home town.
- The fear of gay men being discovered, including a fear of anti-gay violence.
- A critical attitude toward the commercialisation of the gay subculture.
- The lack of bar owners willing to take the economic risk of creating a gay establishment.

As a young man commented,

> Among gay men there is no high regard for a commercial subculture. This attitude needs to change in order to accept that a gay pub is a place of living culture. That attitude is missing among bar owners and their patrons.

In contrast to the rejection of gay pubs in Leipzig, gay men have easily accepted gay saunas. This trend is supported by the closing of public restrooms and their being replaced by automated toilets. Older men are particularly disadvantaged by this development because they can be reluctant to go into the youth-dominated saunas because of their age and because the saunas have different rituals for making contact.

Regarding changes in the gay subculture, the maxim for Rostock (a city on the Baltic Sea which in 1996 had 231,300 residents) is 'Now after ten years nothing has changed in this respect'. One activist in Rostock commented concerning the development of the gay subculture:

> We've looked around in the West and we've tried to install a commercial gay scene. [. . .] But I think it's going to stay like it is for the foreseeable future. [. . .] I thought the fall of the Wall would change everything [but] it didn't change anything in regard to this issue.

This statement supports the notion that the adoption of western-style gay subcultures – even in larger cities – will not occur until gay men who underwent western socialisation play the major role in the gay scene. Rostock had a gay beach, making it a favourite vacation destination for gay men from throughout Eastern Europe. The city also had a gay group founded by activists in the mid-1980s. Since the lifting of travel restrictions, the beach has lost its draw for gay tourists. The gay group, like many in East Germany, is attended largely by men who were socialised under the former government, conditions which the younger generation of gay men never experienced. This has led to a generation conflict found throughout the East, creating the necessity for generation-specific HIV prevention.

Hoyerswerda, a city located in the far eastern part of the country, was once an important centre for the coal industry. Since the Wall fell, the industry has been shut down, with no other employers to take its place. Today, the city has an unemployment rate of 24.1 per cent, one of the highest in Germany (per the Employment Office in Hoyerswerda as of December 1997). In connection to the worsening social conditions in recent years, several xenophobic attacks against foreigners have occurred; however, a subject there said during his interview 'I have not heard that there is violence against gays'. In the typical East German industrial city gay men were invisible. Whereas it posed no problem to find interview partners in other cities, it was very difficult in Hoyerswerda. A representative of the gay group there reported that the men place a great deal of value in anonymity and not calling attention to themselves. 'Feminine' acting men are rejected. There are no public sexual meeting places, private networks being most important. In addition, gay men prefer to go to Dresden or to East Berlin to meet their sexual needs. Because of this situation it is no wonder that there have been no violent assaults of gay men there; the gay men are unrecognisable as such.

A gay activist in the famous historical town of Quedlinburg (25,478 residents in 1995) says 'Today I have to be more concerned about my reputation'. To explain he added,

> Some people wonder if they should be seen on the street with me. That is a real small-minded sort of set back. This isn't exactly anti-gay. Today we're in a pushy society in which discrediting others plays a central role in order to make things better for yourself.

This comment illustrates the effect of the changing social climate and the new prejudices for gay men in the eastern part of the country. If gay men are invisible in their home towns like in Quedlinburg or Hoyerswerda, then violence against them cannot occur.

The motto for Zittau (population 38,144 in 1988, decreasing to 29,000 in 1995 due to emigration from the city) is 'The walls are growing'. This is in reference to the increasing influence of socio-economic status on the coherence and composition of networks of friends. These networks were of great importance in East Germany because of the lack of a gay subculture as part of public life. Social disadvantage played very little role. These networks have undergone dramatic shifts, however, caused by the emigration of eastern gays to the West and social pressures to associate in different ways, for example by social status. The context from which the above quoted statement originates is,

> Those who became rich after the Wall fell [that is, those who maintained their job or who found a new line of work] try to overlook that I'm unemployed. But it's then that a new wall is built up, a wall that no one wants, a wall that no one can do anything about.

The changes in the gay subculture in eastern Germany since 1989 are very diverse. Table 13.3 to 13.6 present selected aspects of these changes.

These tables show that, just as the biographies of individual men have undergone transformation, interruption and confrontation with the new state of affairs since the Wall fell, collective gay life has also changed. There has been a marked growth in collective forms of gay life, the extent of which is beyond the scope of this study. At the same time it is surprising how much continuity one finds, at both the individual and collective level. This is a sign that forty years of separation led to the development of different social forms in the two Germanys, not only in regard to gay life. Ten years after the Wall there remain important differences between the subcultures in East and West. These differences will likely remain until gay men socialised after reunification begin to play a more important role in determining the structures of gay life. These differences continue to be relevant for HIV prevention, as well, although they have been nearly completely ignored. The differing attitudes toward the disease and toward risk, as well as the differing forms of socialising and the associated communication structures and approaches to life have not been taken into account. A new

Table 13.3 Trends in the gay subculture in eastern Germany: organisations and groups (public sphere)

	Tasks and functions	*Social importance since unification*	*Group membership*
Groups existing prior to 1989 in East Germany which have essentially continued unchanged (e.g., as in Leipzig)	Sense of security Solidarity Information Education Counselling	Decreasing	Men who came out before 1989
Groups existing prior to 1989 in East Germany which have changed since unification, offering discos, semi-commercial venues (e.g., as in Rostock)	Cultural and leisure activities Solidarity Finding sex-partners	Increasing	Both men who came out before and who came out after 1989
Groups founded after 1989 *a) Groups within (multi-) cultural centres (e.g, as in Quedlinburg and Zittau)*	Cultural and leisure activities Socialising Counselling	Slightly increasing	Men who came out after 1989 and men of various sexual orientations
b) Groups based on Western models (e.g., as in Leipzig)	Religious, political, cultural and sports activities	Increasing	Men who came out after 1989 Men who migrated from western to eastern Germany

Note: The Berlin Wall fell in 1989

Table 13.4 Trends in the gay subculture in eastern Germany: commercial establishments (public sphere)

	Tasks and functions	*Social importance since unification*	*Group membership*
Gay pubs, bars, cafes, etc.	Socialising Finding sex partners	Unimportant in small towns (very few in existence)	Mainly men who came out before 1989
		Increasing inportance in larger cities, drawing men from the entire region on weekends; bars and clubs opened after 1989 prefered.	Mainly men who came out after 1989
Mixed Pubs (gay, lesbian, heterosexual)	Socialising Finding sex partners	Consistently important, both before and after unification	Mixed ages Gay men without strong subcultural affiliation
Gay discos	Entertainment Socialising	Increasing	Mainly younger gay men who came out after 1989
Gay saunas	Sex contacts	Increasing	Mainly younger gay men (to 40 years old)

prevention concept needs to be developed based on the social reality of gay men in eastern Germany, with the form and content of the strategy being adapted to the regional attitudes and experience. (See also Rosenbrock, 1994.)

Improving HIV prevention for east German gay men

Tables 13.7 to 13.9 summarise the prevention needs of gay men and ways in which current approaches could be adapted to better meet these needs.

As the tables indicate, the most important recommendation for improving

Table 13.5 Trends in the gay subculture in eastern Germany: locations for sexual encounters (public sphere)

	Tasks and functions	*Social importance since unification*	*Group membership*
Public toilets (cottages) and their surroundings	Sex contacts Socialising	Clearly decreasing due to facilities being replaced by automatic toilets	Mainly older gay men (over 40 years old)
Cruising areas (parks, beaches)	Sex contacts Socialising	Slightly decreasing	Mixed ages

Table 13.6 Trends in the gay subculture in eastern Germany: personal life (private sphere)

	Tasks and functions	Social importance since unification	Group membership
Networks of friends	Social stability Leisure time Socialising	Strongly decreasing due to migration to the West and to larger cities and due to the growing influence of income, education and social status on socialising	Mainly gay men who came out before 1989
Sexual Networks	Sexual contacts Socialising	Slightly decreasing	Mixed ages

prevention in eastern Germany concerns how the information is communicated to the target group. Since 1992 there has been a stagnation in the founding of new AIDS Service Organisations (ASOs) in the eastern part of the country due to the low number of infected persons there as well as to the emigration of people with HIV/AIDS to the larger cities. Therefore, it would be useful to promote a greater integration of existing gay organisations into the activities of the public health authorities. Such a collaboration can only be possible if both paid and volunteer staff of gay organisations receive further training in prevention work. The

Table 13.7 Challenges in HIV prevention for gay men in eastern Germany: agents of prevention

	Description of problem	Proposed solution
Local AIDS Service Organisations (ASOs)	Lack of contact with the gay subculture	Integration of ASOs in the structures of the subculture
	Lack of outreach	Development of outreach programmes in places where gay men meet
Gay Organisations	Lack of participation in prevention activities	Raising awareness in these organisations about the need for prevention
	Lack of volunteer training	Training programmes specific to prevention activities
	Lacking financial support	Funding from public authorities
Public Health Departments	Professionally questionable attitudes concerning HIV tests (e.g., recommending all gay men be tested)	Further education for staff regarding HIV testing
	Discrimination against gay men. Prejudices regarding self-help structures	Increasing support for alternative prevention measures; education on the diversity of gay lifestyles

Table 13.8 Challenges in HIV prevention for gay men in eastern Germany: methods of prevention

	Description of problem	Proposed solution
Educational/ Informational Events for gay groups	Rapidly growing lack of interest; however, information level of group members high	Focus on negotiation and interpersonal communication skills regarding safer sex
Counselling (In-person and by Telephone)	Lack of trained personnel within gay organisations	Training for volunteers within gay organisations
Printed Material	Growing lack of interest	Research to describe the role of printed material and the value of various content
	Lack of authenticity of explicit materials designed for gay men	Socially and culturally adapted printed material
	Lack of locations for distributing explicitly gay material	Focus on strengthening interpersonal skills as opposed to location-specific themes
	Lack of readiness on the part of gay pub owners to display material	Raising the awareness of pub owners regarding the need for prevention
Outreach Work	Occurring less frequently due to reduced funding and a lack of awareness on the part of the agents of prevention regarding the need for outreach	Raising awareness within the ASOs and the public authorities regarding the need for outreach
Peer Group Involvement	Lack of models for recruiting and training gay volunteers	Developing models for the design and implementation of peer-based work
TV advertisements	No content related to gay life in rural areas and small towns	Production of ads reflecting the lifestyles of men outside of large cities

existing AIDS Service Organisations should also attempt to build stronger ties to the gay subculture, as many ASOs in the western part of the country have done. In this way, the ASOs can establish their role as advocates for gay men.

At the methodological level there is an urgent need for strengthening outreach-oriented approaches (for example, outreach workers in the gay scene and peer involvement). The prevention messages themselves should take into account the contradictions and the problematic elements of prevention strategies which exist in light of the unique history of this part of the country. Up to this point, these difficulties have been largely overlooked or ignored.

Conclusion

The research questions posed at the beginning of this chapter asking whether or not the prevention concepts from West Germany were successful when applied to

Table 13.9 Challenges in HIV prevention for gay men in eastern Germany: content of prevention messages

	Description of problem	Proposed solution
Needs of the target group	Current focus on gay men in cities where no ASO present	Involvement of gay organisations in prevention which are located in smaller cities and town
Consistency of messages	Historical contradictions between messages in East and West Germany	Making the contradictions between the messages of the two former countries clear through media campaigns and promoting dialogue
The role of medical interventions	Focus on HIV test as prevention, particularly within medical institutions; relegating resposibility for prevention to the medical establishment	Education emphasising the need for personal responsibility in risk-taking
The visibility of AIDS	Perception of eastern Germany as being an 'epidemiological island', reinforced by the migration of people with HIV/ AIDS to larger cities	Information and education promoting a climate of social acceptance for people with HIV/AIDS
Selection of sex partner	Selecting partner based on whether he is 'known' or 'unknown' to the individual or the network	Education regarding the risks of this strategy while promoting safer sex as preferable to partner selection

the East German context cannot be answered with a simple yes or no. In general, one can say that the concepts have had success in preventing widespread epidemic; however, when examining in greater detail how men have responded to these concepts, as we have done here, the deficits become apparent. The success of HIV prevention in eastern Germany could have been greater if the specific social and historical characteristics of this part of the country had been taken more into account. In doing the latter, stabilisation of the epidemic over the longer term will be possible. Therefore, existing prevention strategies need to be improved in order to best meet the needs of eastern German gay men.

Acknowledgements

Many thanks to Robert Kohler, Wilhelm Werthern and Brian Currid for their comments.

Note

1   East Berlin, the former capital of East Germany, is an exception to many of the epidemiological trends found in other parts of the eastern region, given that it is now a part of the united Berlin. This has generally meant a more marked westernisation of all aspects of life, including gay culture.

References

Bochow, M. (1993) 'Reactions of the gay community to AIDS in East and West Berlin', in *Deutsche AIDS-Hilfe* (ed.), *Aspects of AIDS and AIDS-Hilfe in Germany, AIDS-Forum* vol. XII, Berlin: Deutsche AIDS-Hilfe.

—— (1997) *Schwule Männer und AIDS, AIDS-Forum* vol. XXXI, Berlin: Deutsche AIDS-Hilfe.

Herrn, R. (1999) *Schwule Lebenswelten im Osten: andere Orte, andere Biographien, AIDS-Forum* vol. XXXIV, Berlin: Deutsche AIDS-Hilfe.

Reisbeck, G., Edinger, M., Junker, H., Keupp, H. and Knoll, C. (1993) 'Soziale Netzwerke schwuler Männer im Zeichen von AIDS' in Cornelia Lange (ed.), *AIDS – eine Forschungsbilanz*, Berlin: edition sigma: 129–38.

Rosenbrock, R. (1994) *Ein Grundriß wirksamer AIDS-Prävention. Zeitschrift für Gesundheitswissenschaften/Journal of Public Health,* 2.3: 233–44.

Rosenbrock, R., Dubois-Arber, F., Moers, M., Pinell, P., Schaeffer, D. and Setbon, M. (1999) *The Normalisation of AIDS in Western European Countries: Social Science and Medicine* (in press).

Strauss, A. L. and Corbin, J. (1996) *Grounded Theory: Grundlagen qualitativer Sozialforschung*, Weinheim: Belz.

14 The accepting approach to working with drug users in Germany

An overview of principles, goals and methods

Gundula Barsch

The AIDS crisis: working with drug users under pressure to modernise

Already in the mid-1980s the necessary structural changes were being discussed in Germany regarding society's approach to drug problems, however this effort was lacking a political push. It took the realisation that users of illegal drugs constituted the second largest population infected with HIV for support to materialise. The reason for this reaction was the fear that this group could infect members of the general population by way of sharing infected needles, prostitution, and transmitting the disease to their regular sexual partners. The result was a new social climate in which a paradigm change regarding drug use was at least tolerated. This provided an opportunity for strategies which rejected the traditional abstinence and 'hitting bottom' approaches to focus on harm reduction by offering social services to address basic needs, drug substitution treatment, and information about techniques for minimising risk (safer use).[1]

An accepting approach in the process of professionalisation

An accepting stance in the work with drug users has gained a decade of practical and political experience. This approach, characterised by harm reduction, is based on pragmatism and integration. This includes offering outreach-based services and accepting drug use as a part of the clients' lifestyle. This approach is in contrast to drug treatment services which demand from their clients abstinence and a motivation to change. An accepting stance also opposes repressive political measures in response to the use of illegal drugs, for example, the criminalisation of users.

The basis for a new concept in drug work: viewing drug use differently

The new concept for drug work rejects a rigid categorising of substance use into dependence and addition. The path from drug use to compulsive and excessive forms of consumption including dependence (whether labelled as such by the social environment or by the user) can take on myriad forms, as can the lifestyle which develops around the use of drugs. Even in the case of 'substance use disorders' in the classical sense, an accepting approach is appropriate. The concrete details of the approach are defined by the specific situation and the resources of the particular client. A mechanistic view which describes the stereotypical physical and psychological consequences of drug use is not viewed as appropriate. Programmes which work according to this view are not able to address the real needs for support and concrete assistance as experienced by drug users.

In addition to the dynamic of the drug using itself, which plays a key role in determining the need for assistance, the unique aspects of the client's situation need to be taken into account which are related to his/her social situation and personal history. This includes: age; gender; socio-economic background; family situation; education; vocational training and experience; the circumstances and timeline related to first drug use; how long the drug has been used compulsively and excessively; the degree of integration in the drug scene; the form and intensity of drug-free contacts; the changing motivation for drug use; the psycho-social meaning of drug use; the length of clean phases (whether self-induced or imposed by others); the length of phases characterised by controlled, pleasurable use; the type of drug used and the way in which it is used; and the conscientious application of risk management regarding frequency, mode, and amount of use. All of these characteristics are important in order to determine the dynamic and the breadth of development regarding one's drug use. As is clear from this list, very different support services are needed depending on the specific situation of the client. In addition, the quality of these services needs to be evaluated and assured.

The main idea behind acceptance: the individual's right to self determination

The cornerstone of an accepting approach is the belief that drug users are able to assume responsibility for their own actions and that they are able to self-determine their own lives. This implies that drug users have the right to being treated with human dignity. This belief is the basis for the principles and goals which have been formulated to guide the performance of work based on acceptance. The following is excerpted from '*Guidelines for an Accepting Approach in Work with Drug Users*' issued by the group *akzept*, the National German Association for an Accepting Approach in Work with Drug Users and a Humane Drug Policy.[2]

The principles for an accepting approach in work with drug users

> Principle 1: acceptance of the drug user as a competent person able to take responsibility for his/her actions and to self-determine his/her life. The drug user has a right to independence and autonomy.

This principle explicitly excludes an authoritative requirement for abstinence as well as the demand for immediate behaviour change. In contrast, the various lifestyles associated with drug use need to be accepted, self-determined life choices need to be supported, and the staff and client need to work together to explore the options to enable a way of dealing with drugs which encourages personal responsibility, minimising risk and achieving pleasure from the use. For some clients this can mean continued drug use, for another a life without drugs. This form of goal-setting is greatly hindered by the general tendency to pathologise the consumers of illegal drugs, to subject them to the client or patient status, and to exclude particular groups of drug users from services.

This focus on personal responsibility and autonomy does not mean that users should be left alone in crisis situations. In contrast to the 'classical' understanding of how best to assist drug users, this principle foresees making decisions on behalf of the user in exceptional situations only.

Principle 2: protecting and defending the human dignity of clients.

Protecting the human dignity of a client is an inviolable tenet of an accepting stance. People using illegal drugs find themselves in a unique situation in society, characterised by policing measures, pressures to abstain from use, and a lack of assistance when suffering from the consequences of use. For this reason it is essential that the human dignity of drug users be defended. An accepting stance explicitly distances itself from such measures as inspections of personal possessions, the collection of urine samples under observation, bathroom stalls which cannot be closed for privacy, the prohibition of sexual contact, the separation of parents from their children, and the overt or often subtle censure of homosexuality.

All work with drug users necessarily involves confrontations with legal sanctions and society's expectations to which staff need to respond. This response should never, however, be at the expense of the client. That is, staff of drug agencies should not understand their role as being paternalistic. In addition, human dignity implies responding to the specifics of the individual's situation.

Principle 3: normalisation of the drug problem and of the status of drug users in society.

The way in which society deals with drugs and drug users is one of the causes of today's drug problems. The use of drugs is most often seen as a 'deviant' behaviour. This results in drug users being required to label themselves as 'failures' in order to receive help and to their being required to take on goals imposed on them by others (for example, abstinence). This dynamic is a barrier to potential clients' making use of available services. In light of this, an accepting approach has a particular ethical responsibility. Changing society's reaction to drugs and drug users is an important goal of an accepting approach, as such change is a precondition for humane and effective social and health care services for this population.

In addition, the network of drug agencies should not become a ghetto for drug users. Integration in existing social and medical assistance structures is therefore an absolutely necessary aspect of an accepting approach.

Principle 4: protecting clients from harm to their health and social well-being, from social stigma, and from criminalisation.

The society's reaction to drug users and drugs often leads to health and social problems for users and provokes negative reactions in the user's social environment (for example, discrimination and persecution). The accepting approach attempts to lessen these negative effects and to counteract a process of self harm. This requires a preventive focus in working with users in which harm reduction has precedent over services to repair the damage already done. All approaches which make use of an individual's 'hitting bottom' in order to motivate change are contrary to the principle described here. In addition, clients must not be harmed by services provided (for example, substitution, detoxification, inpatient treatment, and crisis intervention).

Principle 5: focusing on the needs of clients.

At both the theoretical and practical level, the work with clients is focused on their needs. This does not mean, however, that service providers must respond to all client demands. The support from a provider is the result of a negotiation process between the worker and the client based on goal-setting and weighing the appropriateness of the client's requests. This negotiation process also entails a systematic collaboration with self-help groups and other representatives of clients' interests. The provider of services to drug users is always in service of several funding bodies with varying interests. It is the duty of staff, however, to advocate staunchly for the interests of their clients, analogous to the way in which labour unions act on behalf of their members.

Principle 6: political action concerning drug policy.

An accepting approach to working with drug users requires political action in the interest of change in public policy related to social welfare, health care and drugs with the goal of promoting the principles outlined here. This includes especially the normalisation of drug problems and of the status of drug users in society. Normalisation itself is based on the observation that psychoactive substances (for example, in the form of alcohol, cigarettes, coffee, pills of all sorts) are already an integral part of social norms, used to control and influence our awareness of the environment and our emotional states. Given that the use of such substances is in this sense already 'normal', it should be dealt with in as pragmatic a way as possible. (For a discussion of the concept of normalisation and drug policy see Engelsmann, 1989, and van de Wijngaart, 1991.)

The advantage of normalisation is that it expands the possibilities for how providers of drug services establish contact and work with clients:

- Services are used earlier in a drug-using career before harm has resulted.
- The social integration of the drug user, included integration in a work environment, is more likely.
- Establishing connections with other social service organisations is easier for clients.
- An informed public is less likely to stigmatise drug users and is therefore more likely to show support and tolerance for people with drug problems.

The goals of an accepting approach in work with drug users

Goal 1: the prevention and minimisation of the physical, psychological, and social harm which can result from the use of illegal drugs. This includes making available to drug users the assistance necessary in order to survive and work through problems related to use.

Harm reduction is promoted through providing information about lower risk forms of drug use and safer use practices for injecting drugs as well as through distributing clean needles. Problem-focused assistance is offered through crisis intervention and services to address basic needs.

Goal 2: promoting and improving the health of clients and stabilising their psychosocial situation.

Physical harm resulting from the use of drugs should be prevented or at least minimised. Particularly drug dependence or the excessive use of drugs can impede daily social functioning. Therefore, services for drug users need to address basic day-to-day needs. For example, services which promote personal care and suitable structures for work and leisure activities enable the client to be socially integrated, thus avoiding isolation and marginalisation.

Goal 3: promoting self determination and the potential for self-help.

All services must have the goal of enabling clients to assume responsibility for their own lives through self determination. This is particularly important for forms of drug use whose risk can be minimised so as to reduce the potential of harm to the user and to others. Likewise, services should promote users' making active use of assistance for problems related to using.

Goal 4: promoting social integration and behavioural competency.

Anyone who is discriminated against or stigmatised is not fully able to maintain or develop the skills necessary to perform effectively the tasks of daily living. As a result, social disintegration and isolation are intensified. Particularly the compulsive use of drugs makes coping with daily life difficult, leading to the potential loss of the skills necessary to maintain social integration.

An accepting approach to working with drug users must take into account the social environment of clients when defining service concepts. Strategies should respect the cultural identity and individual lifestyle of the client while securing and expanding the skills necessary to regain the client's participation in the social and cultural life of the community. Above all, the emphasis needs to be placed on achieving integration where the client lives in terms of his/her personal care, work life, family, and in terms of other social contacts. Services need to take into account that clients' skills in these areas may be limited for a considerable period of time.

Methods for an accepting approach in the work with drug users

At first glance the methods described here seem to differ little from traditional ways of working with drug users. The essential character of an accepting approach is not to be found in any specific method, but rather in the full picture of how the various methods are employed in conjunction with one another.

Method 1: focus on the individual.

All services are to be tailored to the individual client. This includes paying careful attention to the varied experiences and needs which can be found among drug users.

Method 2: promoting the quality of the helping relationship.

Drug-related problems can only be addressed where there is mutual respect between the client and the worker. In order to achieve this, a system of helping relationships needs to be established with the client as early as possible. Ideally, every client should work with the same staff person over the longer term and through all phases of the work. This aim should not, however, prevent other professionals with specialised knowledge and skills or other co-operating providers from being including in the helping process.

The helping relationship comprises several aspects:

- Accepting the client for who he/she is without seeing him/her as a 'symptom carrier'.
- Being present to the client as an agent of personal reflection as opposed to just a staff person in the 'function of helper'.
- Being authentic, as appropriate, without being domineering.
- Striking a balance between intimacy and distance based on mutual acceptance, thus avoiding over-identification and merging with the client.

Method 3: transparency in the planning of services.

The planning of services is a co-operative, open process in which all parties (staff and client) are obliged to participate. The client, however, is the focus of this process. Particularly longer-term services need be transparent for both staff and clients so that the work will be coherent, predictable, and open to scrutiny.

Method 4: a multi-dimensional understanding of drug use and dependence.

Work with drug users – everything from intake to diagnosis and intervention – is based on a multi-dimensional (that is, holistic) understanding of drug use and drug dependence. This understanding takes into account the physical, pharmacological, biochemical, psychological, biographical, social and cultural aspects of the aetiology, course, treatment and prognosis of drug problems. Therefore a multi-disciplinary team is necessary in order to achieve the highest quality work in this area.

Method 5: diagnosis (exploration).

Diagnosis is not an end in itself, but rather a tool in service planning which helps to clarify the resources available to the client. Understood in this way, diagnosis is an important element in the professional practice of an accepting approach in the work with drug users.

Each diagnosis needs to relate directly to the various dimensions of the client's life. Current limitations and potential risks need to be determined regarding the client's physical, psychological, and social situation. The details in each of these problem areas need to be clarified together with the client. Problems related to drug use can only be understood when the social context in which the problems arose is taken into account. Because of this, the diagnostic phase of an accepting approach needs to examine multiple dimensions.

In the case of acute interventions the focus needs to be on relieving the immediate stress of physical, psychological, and social problems, particularly any risk for suicide. However, long-term services must take the entire complex of problems into account.

Method 6: incorporating research findings on practice methodology.

Research on the ongoing development of drug use in society is indispensable in order to react appropriately to changes in drug use patterns and in the composition of the drug scene. Where knowledge is lacking or current knowledge has no clear implications for practice, the work with drug users should be conducted according to a professional consensus based on practical experience. In future research it will be increasingly important to incorporate practice-relevant dimensions in study designs.

Method 7: networking among professional groups (multidisciplinary collaboration).

The various professional groups working in the drug field (social workers, sociologists, psychologists, physicians, etc.) and self-help organisations must collaborate so that each can bring its particular perspectives and skills to the work. Multidisciplinary partnerships are a characteristic of professional practice.

Method 8: networking between service providers.

Networking among medical providers, social service providers, and self-help groups – in other words, a co-ordinated collaboration – is an important element of professional care for drug users. This method allows for broadening the spectrum of services, improving access, and preventing a further 'ghettoisation' of drug users within care systems.

Method 9: outpatient over inpatient care.

An accepting approach to work with drug users seeks to offer diagnostic and support services on as much of an outpatient basis as possible. The decision whether or not treatment should be offered inpatient or outpatient should be a mutual one made by staff and clients. Inpatient care is appropriate, at least for a limited period, when it is believed that a certain intervention can only succeed within the protective environment of the inpatient setting.

Method 10: promoting self-help organisations and activities.

An accepting approach to work with drug users seeks to activate the potential for self-help. For this reason, the organisation of self-help groups for users is promoted. This includes providing space and other support so that self-help activities can take place.

Method 11: documentation.

Documentation includes all client information related to diagnosis, care planning, the details of each service offered, and the data necessary for measuring success.

Method 12: confidentiality.

In working with drug users it is important that personal information (for example name, address, age, reason for seeking services) be kept confidential. Lack of care with such data can result in discrimination (for example, being fired from a position). Even the knowledge that someone has had contact with a drug agency can be viewed as a personal deficiency resulting in problems at work and at home.

Method 13: public relations.

Agencies serving drug users need to engage in wide-scale public relations work, providing information about drug use and associated problems as well as about available services for users. This work can ease prejudices and counter fear in society regarding users. In addition, effective public relations efforts can increase the trust which users and non-users have in the work of drug agencies and augment their professional recognition.

Public relations in this sense includes:

- Providing information about the effects of drugs, the ways in which they are used, and the risks involved.
- Debunking the myths associated with drugs and drug using.
- Publicising specific models of how individuals can control their own drug use, with the goal of promoting conscientious use instead of fear and repugnance of drugs and drug users.
- Promoting social (as opposed to legal) control mechanisms regarding drug problems in society.

Method 14: reflection.

A continuous process of reflection regarding the work performed is indispensable in the planning and implementation of the various aspects of work with drug users. This includes:

- Examining the theoretical basis for the work, particularly through regular opportunities for continuing education.
- Reflecting on one's own professional conduct, especially through questioning the causes of particular client outcomes. This reflection is possible through discussion of cases with other staff, thereby learning though experience.
- Observing the circumstances related to rare events, either negative (such as suicide attempts or other violent acts) or positive (such as exceptional progress or a self-initiated end to a drug career).
- Discussing issues regularly in teams.
- Networking and collaborating with other organisations.

The basis for a meaningful examination of the work performed is a climate of openness. There should be a common goal of working through weaknesses and mistakes as opposed to covering them up so that the performance of workers can be improved. This process should be accompanied by group supervision led by a professional from outside the agency.[3]

Measuring quality in professional work with drug users

As is clear in the principles, goals, and methods presented above, an accepting approach in the work with drug users has distanced itself from technocratic concepts of quality and quality management (for example, Total Quality Management or TQM) in its development of quality criteria for professional work in this area. It is the belief that such concepts are not appropriate for social work because they tend to advocate for technical procedures as a way to control quality, thereby prohibiting important discussions related to the content of practice.

In contrast to a technical approach, an accepting approach to work with drug users places top priority on the ability of organisations to promote their own development and to structure their internal process in such a way as to take on voluntarily new challenges in the work as they arise. Examples of such challenges are emerging groups of drug users, the dangers of increasing bureaucracy in the work, and changing funding structures at the local level. It is for this reason that drug work in Germany should not be defined through binding practice standards set from above by a panel of experts, as is the case for several areas of medical care. Instead, the further professionalisation of the drug field should be characterised by establishing guidelines for each specific type of service which, in turn, can constitute a basis for the development of quality criteria in each individual setting.

Currently, the existing consensus regarding service structures and the division of labour is being called into question in Germany because of the pressure to cut spending. Central to this dynamic is the debate over the definition of quality in the field of drug work. Unlike in industries where it is relatively easy to determine the signs of quality regarding a specific tangible product, the drug field performs services for which there are no universally valid standards. The discussion to date has revealed less commonality and more divergence in terms of the interests of the various players. This diversity will necessarily require a variety of ways to define quality for the various social work functions. These differences must be laid bare before the next step can be taken toward finding a consensus.

How one understands quality is directly related to one's role within the drug services system:

- For the client, the usefulness of a particular service is primary. This means that the service needs to relevant to the realities of the client's life and therefore able to address specific needs.
- For the professional, it is important that he/she do 'good work'. This refers to work which is performed according to the ethical principles of his/her profession, as well as according to principles of appropriateness. The judgement of how well professional work is performed arises from a discourse with other professionals – for example, in supervision – where one becomes more aware of his/her actions and the circumstances surrounding them.

- For the funder, regardless whether public or private, quality is defined as the most efficient performance of a particular clearly-defined service. The 'level' at which the service should be performed is a matter of negotiation.
- For the politician, quality is defined as usefulness to society, which of course is intricately connected with the institutional interests of the programs involved.

These very different perspectives cannot be harmonised through the creation of an 'objective' standard for quality. The development of quality criteria for the drug field requires a process of negotiation and clarification. Through the realisation of the principles and methods for the accepting approach to work with drug users presented here, it will be possible to strengthen the profile and promote the professionalism of social work in this area. Most important in Germany in this respect has been the work of *akzept* (The National German Association for an Accepting Approach in Work with Drug Users and a Humane Drug Policy), and the Deutsche AIDS-Hilfe (The National German AIDS Organisation). However, all this will only be possible through a process of working things through, together and one step at a time.

Notes

1   'Hitting bottom' refers to the so-called 'Twelve Steps' approach to drug counselling which is found in English-speaking countries, particularly the US, but is not common in Germany. Traditional approaches to drug treatment in Germany are, however, characterised by a focus on abstinence and allowing the drug user to reach a point of destitution as a motivator for change ('hitting bottom' in Twelve Step terms). This focus is similar to that found in Twelve Step programs.
     The most common form of substitution treatment in many countries is methadone maintenance for opiate addicts. There are, however, other drugs which can be prescribed and monitored by physicians in order to stabilise the psychological, social, and medical condition of drug users.
2   A copy of the original guidelines, published in German, is available from the Deutsche AIDS-Hilfe in Berlin under the title: *akzept* (1999) *Leitlinien für akzeptierende Drogenarbeit*, Materialienband 3.
3   Unlike in many countries, supervision has become a specialised profession of its own in Germany. It is increasingly common that organisations in both the for-profit and non-profit sectors seek the services of supervisors in private practice who have been trained specifically in various methods of assisting groups and individuals in assessing their work. These methods include, for example, clinical supervision, coaching, and organisational consulting.

References

akzept (1999) *Leitlinien für akzeptierende Drogenarbeit*, Materialienband 3, Berlin: Deutsche AIDS-Hilfe.
Engelsmann, E. L. (1989) 'Dutch policy on the management of drug-related problems', *British Journal of Addiction* 84: 211–18.
Wijngaart, van de, F. G. (1991) *Competing Perspectives on Drug Use: The Dutch Experience*, Amsterdam: Swets and Zeitlinger.

15 The meaning of HIV prevention in the context of heterosexual relationships

What are women protecting themselves from?

Cornelia Helfferich

Introduction: HIV prevention as a behaviour in context

The research project 'HIV Prevention as a Behaviour in the Context of Women's Sexual Relationships' (Helfferich *et al.*, 1996), commissioned by the German Federal Ministry for Research and Technology, brought two new aspects to the discussion concerning the development of appropriate prevention concepts. The first aspect was a gender-specific perspective in light of the increasing number of women becoming infected with HIV through heterosexual intercourse. (See Marcus, Chapter 3.) The second aspect was the observation that even the most successful campaigns providing information about HIV risk had their limits; the frequency with which higher risk sexual behaviour occurs in spite of partners 'knowing better' is a sign of resistance regarding these campaigns and the need to provide new ways of conducting prevention. The questions underlying the study were: what is the function, meaning and usefulness of risk behaviour? In what context is this behaviour so integrated as to be maintained in spite of knowing the inherent danger involved? Some studies have examined the situational context of risk behaviour and the barriers to communication about HIV (Gerhards and Schmidt, 1992; Ahlemeyer, 1993; see also Ahlemeyer, Chapter 10). Although this work has been able to clarify the dynamics of various forms of sexual encounter, it has not identified the circumstances in which rules of interpersonal interaction take on a subjective relevance. The focus of our work can therefore be described as 'the context of the context', or in other words, exploring factors which mitigate the effects which the relational context has on HIV risk-taking

This focus on the context of HIV risk in the broadest sense takes into account not only the particular relational situation but also the history of the individuals involved as well as societal influences. The latter refers particularly to the various forms of male and female sexuality as well as gender-related behaviour found in specific groups in society. The resulting patterns of meaning and behaviour define sexual risk in ways which are sanctioned by society.

Elias (1980: 230) noted that 'bed and body' have been accorded the status of 'psychological danger zones [. . .] of the highest level' during the process of civilisation. Given that Elias' work appeared before the AIDS epidemic we can gain insight into the diversity of potential risks which are involved in love and sexual relationships over and above HIV; that is, dependence and subservience, the loss of autonomy and control, failure, shame, vulnerability, hurt, abandonment, etc. Some of these risks are important at the beginning of a relationship while others play more of a role later in the process (Compare Bastard *et al.*, 1997.) It is this view of sexual risk in all its diversity which is the basis for our research. Risk management needs to be investigated in terms of sexuality, not sexuality in terms of risk management (Bajos *et al.*, 1997).

Sample and method

The study was retrospective and exploratory, incorporating both qualitative and quantitative components. Forty-one women between the ages of 20 and 35 were recruited from newspaper advertisements in Freiburg (western Germany) and East Berlin (formerly part of East Germany) and administered a semi-structured interview in 1993. Subjects were selected so as to reflect the largest diversity possible regarding partner status, having/not having children, education, profession and age (within the above range). The interview questions covered the topics of relationships, sexuality, contraception and HIV prevention. This qualitative data was analysed in terms of content, semantics and grammar/syntax in order to build a typology of patterns of behaviour and meaning and their associated HIV prevention strategies. The data from the qualitative study were then used in the second phase of the research to develop items for a survey of women in Rostock (eastern Germany) and Freiburg (western Germany) which was administered to a random sample of 918 women.

Two years later the study was replicated for male samples (Fichtner *et al.*, 1997), including thirty-seven qualitative interviews in Freiburg and East Berlin and 739 standardised questionnaires from Freiburg and Rostock. This allowed for a four-pronged total sample including eastern German women, eastern German men, western German women and western German men. In the final analysis, all data were compared on the basis of gender and region of origin. This chapter will focus on presenting the findings from the women's data.

Results of the qualitative data

A pattern for both eastern and western women: disorientation and disconnection

This pattern is characterised by personal histories of suffering with a lack of development of adequate coping strategies. One recurring theme was confusion regarding the outside world (powerlessness, having 'nothing to hold on to', the inexplicability of one's own and others' behaviour, psychological retreat, persistent disparity between one's fantasies and reality, derealisation). Other themes included difficulties in relationships (relationships 'slipping away', inability to maintain consistency in relationships, fear and disgust related to men and sex, sexual compulsivity) and problems maintaining boundaries. Relationships and sexuality were either characterised by dissociation and feelings of estrangement or they were rejected all together through distancing or choosing men as partners who were sexually inhibited.

All of the women in this group took greater risks regarding HIV infection, and they were not consistently aware of the potential consequences of their behaviour. In the few cases where protection was found, it was rather by chance, either due to a fearful avoidance of sexual contact (due to a fear of sex, not a fear of HIV) or as a result of relegating the responsibility to the partner, without communicating this explicitly to him. We believe that the risk-taking of these women can be explained in terms of the priority accorded to HIV risk within the realm of the psychological risks tied to relationships and sexuality in general. As one subject said, the risk for HIV was 'not that important' because 'other things are a lot more difficult to deal with'. This prioritisation of risks means that, for this group of women, protective behaviour and HIV risk are symbolically relevant to the extent that they are connected to the 'other things'. Not only does one find a lack of ability to react effectively in regard to sexual situations and to one's own needs but also the lack of ability to follow through with protective behaviour. The lack of reality-based thinking, lack of cognitive self control, and the experience of being estranged from sexuality promote magical thinking regarding protective measures and thus discourage taking an active role in risk situations. What takes places is not experienced as being the result of one's own actions. The quotation 'I couldn't take care of myself', illustrates this problem at its many levels. Intentional, rationally-based protective strategies are not applicable to this group.

Three patterns found among western German women related to biographical themes

The first pattern has at its core a complex of values – orderliness, security, normality, stability, commitment and mutuality – which are imbedded in the collective value system in which the subject lives. This pattern expresses itself at a subtle level of personal interaction with a focus on creating harmony in situations and reacting in accordance with what is socially desirable. The most common relationship form is a long-term partnership from an early age with a rejection or fear of infidelity and being alone. Sexual desires are secondary.

In relation to AIDS there is a tendency not to take risks and to feel protected by the long-term relationship. AIDS is represented in two ways by women exhibiting this pattern. First, there are women who view the world as being divided into a 'normal, stable family-oriented world' and a contrary world of infidelity, promiscuity, bodily fluids, discos, sexual techniques, irresponsibility, etc. AIDS belongs unquestionably to this latter world. In the cases where a fear of AIDS was expressed it stood for the degree to which the subject's own normality was being threatened by the alternative, negative world, or for the subject's ongoing relationship being threatened by her partner's infidelity. That is, the fear of AIDS had little to do with the actual risk of viral transmission. At the same time, the existence of AIDS was seen as affirming the relationship style of the subject as being prudent because it was protective. Second, HIV prevention came into play under the rubric security, responsibility and strengthening the mutuality in the relationship. Condoms were seen as negative because they 'come in-between' the partners, therefore impeding intimacy; whereas, a joint HIV test secures the basis for the relationship. Condoms were further seen as hurtful in that the partner 'selfishly' protects himself thereby avoiding the issue of a potential pregnancy and an owning up to the relationship. An indicator of mutuality was also trust and the associated ability to delegate responsibility to the partner. In general, behaviour regarding contraception and HIV risk was most consistent among subjects who had the least ambivalence about their protective 'normal world', and who were able to integrate risk situations and issues of protection into that world.

The second pattern is comprised of those interviews which have as a central motif the struggle to find autonomy and to define boundaries for oneself. This struggle involves a process of self-realisation (as opposed to estrangement), the search 'to find out what I want', and discovering, naming, valuing, and actively asserting one's own needs and desires in relationships. To a certain extent the process of self-realisation is tied in with the motif of tension between the genders. Relationships with men are confining, distancing a woman from her own needs, making her a passive object. The relationship histories of these women bear witness to a process of searching in the form of 'trying things out', where one alternates between intimate relationships, emotionally or geographically distant relationships, and periods of being alone. The latter are viewed as being times of 'finding out what I like, who I am', offering a freedom from the constriction and domination – also on the sexual level – found in relationships with men. The establishment of a carefulness in regard to relationships as well as the attempt to choose 'harmless' partners or to reduce the frequency of sexual intercourse can be interpreted as a protection from the most important risk in the relationship, namely, the loss of autonomy.

Women exhibiting this pattern were in search of forms of contraception and HIV prevention which both meet the demands imposed by the partnership and one's own needs and which offer control (the latter particularly important where a negative stance or mistrust toward men was present). Parallel to developments in the areas of partnership and contraception was an increasingly conscious and consistent approach to HIV risk. Insisting on the use of a condom in spontaneous sexual encounters could, for example, be related to the desire to test the reaction of the partner in a provocative way and to assist the women in gaining mastery over the situation. AIDS was also used as a tool for discussing an important issue in the relationship (for example, infidelity), talk of the disease providing the appearance of a rational and emotionally distanced handling of the topic. In general, condoms were seen by these women as being positive in that they function as a way of setting boundaries. However, this position is not without ambivalence. The 'struggle' inherent in preventive measures is extremely draining and is itself constricting in its demand for 'self-discipline' and 'being focused'. There is also an aspect of loss to the extent that control of the risk for infection symbolises control over one's own sexual desires or the desire to merge with one's partner. Because this loss, the risk for HIV resulted in a return to more committed partnerships for some women in the long run, demonstrating the ambivalence in those who fear the loss of autonomy.

A defensive strategy to deal with the psychic risk of losing one's autonomy as well as with the risks for pregnancy and HIV infection for women in this group was the reduction of sexual contacts, particularly intercourse. Here we noticed a melding of the danger of AIDS with the threat posed by sexually-active men. In general the risk for pregnancy was more of a cause for action than AIDS risk. A great deal of anxiety, reaching panic proportions by some, was connected to pregnancy, because this meant repeating the fate of one's mother and thereby losing one's autonomy.

A third pattern found among western German women has to do with self-reflection and the meaning attributed to one's life. A common motif was 'being able to talk about everything'. The central values, reflecting this ability to articulate, are openness, clarity, freedom (from unconscious motives), seriousness, reciprocity, trust, understanding, and mutuality. This pattern has commonalties with the second pattern described above, but is constituted of enough unique elements to be described here separately. For these women – even in partnerships which were established slowly, carefully, and later in life – talking is important. We interpret the meaning of this 'talking about everything' at the beginning of a relationship to be a test whether the partner is serious and can wait or if he is only sexually driven. In general, the women were able to achieve a reciprocity and a slow tempo in sexual relationships. The gradual development of intimacy was emphasised by many subjects, offering an apparent assurance (as compared to a 'surprise attack' style of relating). Through verbal exchange a certain level of negotiation regarding needs could be established to which the partners could react (the verbal exchange perhaps being more effective than the sexual exchange).

Discussion of contraception and HIV prevention was at the same time a discussion about how the couple wants to direct the course of the relationship, including the sexual aspects. Preference was given to forms of risk management which require that the couple 'talk openly about it'. When in doubt, intercourse or even other forms of sexual contact were avoided. Behaviour regarding both forms of risk (pregnancy and HIV infection) is directly related to the view that taking these risks seriously means taking one's partner seriously. Through talking, clarity can be gained as to whether the partner is responsible enough. In relation to HIV risk this means in particular that the partner reveal information about his previous sexual contacts and thereby establish trust. However, apart from this functional approach to risk at the beginning of the relationship, women exhibiting this pattern generally feel protected by their fidelity and carefulness, expecting the same behaviour from their partners as a matter of course.

Two patterns found among eastern German women related to biographical themes

All eastern German subjects were of the opinion that 'there was no AIDS' in East Germany; AIDS could not 'burst through the Wall' (the metaphor of flooding was common in these interviews). East Germany was 'a nice island' where one could 'live without danger'. Before unification AIDS was associated with marginalised groups such as prostitutes, homosexuals and foreigners. After the Wall fell, the security of life in East Germany was lost. In many interviews there was an association between the Wall falling and AIDS risk.

One pattern found among eastern German women is characterised by the themes of carrying on the traditions of their parents: family as an important means of collectively holding people together. The latter includes a collective security and integration in the form of 'acting and being like everyone else'. This means adjusting one's life to meet society's expectations as well as a pragmatic adaptation to the given limitations of any situation. Responsibility, seriousness, honesty, security, groundedness, and a strict up-bringing were positive values which are to be lived out within the family context. The pattern of behaviour concerning partners consisted of entering a partnership early in life with the man to whom they were still married and with whom they had children. The family had a high level of importance and should not be put at stake by infidelity and irresponsible sex. Particularly after the Wall fell, the emphasis was on keeping the family together. Knowing one's partner and sharing a family life with him (as opposed to sexual desire) were primary.

The subjects in this group who were in an ongoing relationship had a feeling of being protected 'in the belief that my husband is faithful', or in the belief that he has a strong sense of responsibility. A strong fear of AIDS made one 'glad' to be 'taken care of', making it unnecessary to deal with the 'complicated questions' concerning protection. And 'what you read about AIDS only makes you more careful'. In the hypothetical case of a spontaneous sexual encounter with another man, the subjects reported that they would hesitate to become involved, choosing to wait or to avoid the sexual contact altogether, consistent with their behaviour in general.

The subjects spoke in a disparaging way both about the threat posed by AIDS and about the changes in sexual morality since the Wall fell. 'AIDS has nothing to do with us; I don't want to know anything more about it'. It was shocking to the women that what used to be taboo and 'risqué', like condoms, were now available to the general public. The motivation for protection in the case of an hypothetical affair is the responsibility for one's partner and the duty to one's children. ('You can't just think about yourself; you also have to protect the family . . . because the family needs me, the children need me.')

A second pattern among eastern German women centres around 'I knew what I wanted': that is, experimenting and action, self-control and self-awareness, as well as wanting to gather experience (wanting to be special). In general this is connected with 'keeping cool' regarding men and with various forms of distancing oneself from the example of one's parents and from the typical life of women under socialism. Experimenting refers to changing partners and ways of performing sex. Among these women are the two interviews in our sample with reports of defined phases of living out one's 'pure sexual desire' without being in a relationship. Curiosity, interest, the desire for knowledge, and the attraction of forbidden fruit are characteristic of these women (which also means not marrying the first one who comes along and 'at the age of twenty-two being barefoot and pregnant'). The partner relationships themselves develop in one of two directions: emphasizing the connection due to having a family together or continuing in the spirit of experimentation. In contrast to the subjects from the West, these women described themselves as the type who always used her head; only in one case was life depicted as a process of learning ('It took me a while to realise what I want and to learn how to articulate that').

Concerning HIV prevention the guiding principle 'I know what I want' took the form of emphasizing 'using your head' in sexual encounters and being cautious, particularly when a man cannot be trusted. Preventive behaviour was related to being active, making things clear, and establishing a 'nice' distance: which makes using condoms no problem. This applies foremost to the early stages of a relationship and to affairs (most of the women were in a long-term relationship having begun before the Wall fell). In spite of the emphasis on the ability to follow through with protection in sexual situations outside of the ongoing partnership, the reports of the women changed after the Wall fell from certainty to conjecture, given that the subjects had little concrete experience with the use of condoms ('Up to this point it's been more of a theoretical issue'). AIDS is an issue for these women as it relates to whether or not one needs to 'become more straight-laced' and regarding the new necessity of needing to trust one's partner and his fidelity or at least his using protection when having sex outside of the relationship. These subjects express that it is appropriate not to let oneself be led by one's feelings but also state that 'without feelings it doesn't work either'.

Results of the quantitative data

The quantitative phase of study allowed for testing the typology which was constructed on the basis of the qualitative data. Items for the questionnaire were created by extracting material from the above named patterns. Through a pre-test, scales representing the central dimensions of the patterns were piloted: orientation to marriage and family, perception of relationships, negativity toward sexuality, sexual communication skills, trust, fear of AIDS and the rejection of condom use.

For the total sample of women, a hierarchical cluster analysis resulted in a three cluster solution for western women and a two cluster solution for eastern women.

The first cluster for western women combines the elements of pattern one (traditional family perspective) and pattern three (talking about the relationship) as described in the presentation of the qualitative data above. This includes an elevated fear of AIDS, negativity toward sexuality, and protection strategies characterised by trusting the partner and talking to him about risks, with condoms viewed as endangering intimacy. The second cluster corresponds to the second pattern for western women described above (autonomy), which includes a critical stance regarding the traditional model of family, a positive stance toward sexuality and condoms, and a readiness to confront the issue of AIDS. In this second cluster we found predominantly women with a higher level of education. The third cluster, consisting of elements from the autonomy pattern with an emphasis on aspects of control, appears to correspond to the pattern of disorientation and disconnection found in the qualitative data for both western and eastern women. This cluster combines a defensiveness and a negativity regarding sexuality, a distrust of men, difficulty maintaining relationships, difficulty communicating sexual desires, and a lower fear of AIDS related to an infrequency of sexual contact to men.

For the eastern sample, the first cluster includes a less negative view of sexuality, a somewhat elevated orientation toward family, a higher level of skill in sexual communication, less of a tendency to reject condoms, and a less pronounced fear of AIDS. Women in this cluster tend also to be better educated. The second cluster consists of more negativity toward sexuality, a weaker orientation toward family, less skill regarding sexual communication, a lesser fear of AIDS, and less rejection of condoms. In contrast to the western subjects, the clusters here differ from each other regarding the desire to manage contraception on one's own, which is found more strongly among the women (in cluster one) who are more strongly family oriented. This is so because in East Germany contraception has traditionally been part of the woman's role. The two clusters for eastern women do, indeed, identify two distinct groups; however, the patterns described within the qualitative data could not be replicated. The latter may be due to methodological problems. Firstly, it was difficult to formulate items and scales with an equal validity for both East and West. Secondly, for eastern women it is less difficult to separate items related to a family orientation (which is generally high for the eastern sample) from items related to an assertion of one's self-interest, as the latter was an integral part of the image for all women within socialism.

Discussion

For both eastern and western Germany patterns could be identified related to specific risks associated with heterosexual relationships. The importance of one's personal history regarding such risks had been identified previously in a French study (Bajos *et al.*, 1997). The discussion here reflects other typologies related to social class and gender role which have been proposed. (Compare Koppetsch and Burkart, 1999; and concerning relationship styles, Fichtner, 1999.)

HIV prevention behaviour can be interpreted within the context of the patterns identified here, the behaviour variously related to reducing fear, having control over a situation, affirming the normality of one's behaviour, etc. The logic of preventive behaviour is less a product of a rational decision to avoid illness and more the result of how the psychological risks inherent in heterosexual relationships are managed. Although preventive behaviour cannot be described as rational, it is also not an irrational act. (Compare Reimann and Bardeleben, 1992.) The stronger the psychological threat posed by sexuality, men, and relationships in general, and the more disconnection and disorientation one experiences related to such situations, the more difficult it is to practice a consistent and rational prevention strategy. In our descriptions of the patterns above, we suggested ways of understanding characteristic responses to subjectively relevant forms of risk in sexual relationships in general, and to the associated HIV prevention strategies in particular. Here East and West will be compared in the interest of discussing the meaning of risk perception in the two groups.

An orientation toward normality and family values was found in both parts of the country with characteristic differences regarding what is meant by 'normal' and 'family' in the East and West. The loss of autonomy as a central risk in intimate relationships was important for a subgroup of western women. For them, there is a characteristic search for a balance between intimacy and distance, autonomy and mutuality, and the associated forms of HIV prevention and contraception, including verbal negotiation and a confrontational boundary setting with men. The eastern counterpart to these women already 'knows what she wants' and uses more pragmatic, pleasure-seeking, and less negotiated strategies, without calling these into question. In general, the women from the East felt more self-assured and less dependent on their partners. This difference can be attributed to the economic independence of women in the former East Germany, with most mothers working while raising children. (Compare Begenau and Helfferich, 1997.) Comparison of the social systems in the former East and West Germany also show that whereas the antagonism between the genders in the private sphere was the constitutive element for gender relations in the West, it was the antagonism between the unifying family versus the State which was decisive in the East (Engler, 1992). Family and commitment in a relationship are seen as threats to autonomy in the West; whereas, in the East the family was the means of limiting the scope of the State's influence in one's life as well as a guarantee for an independent provision of material goods. This difference between East and West is also reflected in the ways in which young women in the two parts of the country go about leaving their families of origin to establish their own lives. Not only the psychological risks but also the forms of risk management are different for western and eastern women. In the West one finds verbal strategies of self-assertion as a counterpoint to Christian sexual morals; in the East it is pragmatic decision-making and action juxtaposed with a socialist sexual moral code. The motivations for HIV prevention likewise are different in East and West, reflecting the overall risk management context.

The most important difference between East and West can be found in the statement that in East Germany 'there was no AIDS'. This has meant that a confrontation with AIDS is connected to a confrontation with the new freedoms and threats since unification. (Compare Herrn, Chapter 13.) For conservatives, the fall of the Wall requires families to hold together, shutting out AIDS completely. For others, the frustration and insecurities related to HIV prevention and AIDS are part and parcel of the radical new orientation which unification has demanded of them.

It became clear during the study that AIDS can stand for many things; for example, a feared infidelity and a subversive promiscuity, for the fall of the Wall and the resultant changes, or for a confirmation of one's life choices. One's awareness of AIDS is likewise coloured by the threats with which it is symbolically associated. It also became clear that a manipulation of how one perceives AIDS – whether through dramatising or playing down the danger – has its usefulness; for example, to legitimise one's current prevention strategy, to relieve anxiety, etc. In the narratives, the comments concerning the fear of AIDS were not totally consistent, but rather, they changed in accordance with the thematic content of the interview. Therefore, we can surmise that one's perception of AIDS (whether fearful or otherwise) is not only a factor influencing one's behaviour, for example, by serving as a basis for demanding fidelity in a relationship and limiting sexual contacts. Perception can also be used as a way to circumvent risk, accompanied by forms of behaviours and relationship which are in response to the psychological risks of sexuality. The relationship between perception and behaviour is more complex than linear causality, indicating the existence of personal risk constructions.

In the quantitative phase of the study we were able to confirm through a cluster analysis the patterns identified within the qualitative data for western women. In the East, two groups were found: a more distressed group and a more 'capable' group. Methodological problems arose in that items which are the basis for pattern differences in the West (such as orientation to family) are less able to distinguish between groups of eastern women. More research is needed which uses a larger sample to examine the effects of personal history and the social and cultural context in the two regions. (Compare Bajos *et al.*, 1997.)

The basic idea that HIV prevention is to be understood within the context of how risks are managed in general has been shown to be of importance. This analysis offers relevant target group specific characteristics which can serve as the basis for prevention messages, taking into account the particular types of resistance and patterns of logic found in certain groups of women.

References

Ahlemeyer, H. W. (1993) 'Aidsprävention als Systemintervention: Konturen des Zusammenhangs von intimer Kommunikation und HIV-Risiko-Management', in C. Lange (ed.), *Aids – Eine Forschungsbilanz*, Berlin: edition sigma: 197–210.

Bajos, N., Ducot, B., Spencer, B., Spira, A. and ACSF-Group (1997) 'Sexual risk-taking, socio-sexual biographies and sexual interaction: elements of the French National Survey on Sexual Behaviour', *Social Science and Medicine* 44(1): 25–40.

Bastard, B., Carida-Vonèche, L., Peto, D. and Campenhoudt, L. (1997) 'Relationships between sexual partners and ways of adapting to the risk of AIDS: Landmarks for a relationship-oriented conceptual framework', in L. Campenhoudt, M. Cohen, G.

Guizzardi and D. Hausser (eds), *Sexual Interactions and HIV Risk*, London: Taylor and Francis: 44–59.

Begenau, J. and Helfferich, C. (1997) 'Kinder oder keine? Zu Kontrazeption, Schwangerschaftsabbrüchen und Familienplanung in Ost- und Westdeutschland', in J. Begenau and C. Helfferich (eds), *Frauen in Ost und West – zwei Kulturen, zwei Gesellschaften, zwei Gesundheiten?* Freiburg: Jos Fritz Verlag: 32–59.

Elias, N. (1980) *Über den Prozeß der Zivilisation. Soziogenetische und psychogenetische Untersuchungen. Bd. 1*, Frankfurt/M.: Suhrkamp, 7. Aufl.

Engler, W. (1992) 'Individualisierung im Staatssozialismus' in B. Schäfers (ed.) *Lebensverhältnisse und soziale Konflikte im neuen Europa*. Verhandlungen des 26. Deutschen Soziologentages in Düsseldorf 1992, Frankfurt/Main: Campus: 185-93.

Fichtner, J. (1999) *Über Männer und Verhütung. Der Sinn kontrazeptiver Praxis für Partnerschaftsssstile und Geschlechterverhältnis*, Münster: Waxmann.

Fichtner, J., Helfferich, C., Schehr, K. and Weise, E. (1997) *HIV-Schutz und Kontrazeption als sinnhaftes Handeln von Männern. Eine qualitative und quantitative Erhebung. Abschlußbericht im Auftrag des Bundesministeriums für Forschung und Technologie*, Freiburg: Abteilung für Med, Soziologie der Universität Freiburg.

Gerhard, J. and Schmidt, B. (1992) *Intime Kommunikation. Eine empirische Studie über Wege der Annäherung und Hindernisse für 'safer sex'*, Baden-Baden: Nomos.

Helfferich, C., Schehr, K. and Weise, E. (1996) *HIV-Schutz und Kontrazeption als sinnhaftes Handeln von Frauen. Eine qualitative und quantitative Erhebung. Abschlußbericht im Auftrag des Bundesministeriums für Forschung und Technologie*, Freiburg: Abteilung für Med. Soziologie der Universität Freiburg.

Koppetsch, C. and Burkart, G. (1999) *Die Illusion der Emanzipation. Zur Wirksamkeit latenter Geschlechtsnormen im Milieuvergleich*, Konstanz: Universitätsverlag.

Reimann, B. W. and Bardeleben, H. (1992) *Permissive Sexualität und präventives Verhalten. Ergebnisse einer Untersuchung an Studierenden*, Berlin: edition sigma.

16 The Umbrella Network

AIDS, STD prevention, and prostitution on the eastern border of Germany

Elfriede Steffan and Michael F. Kraus

Background

Europe has grown into a community embracing a wide range of political, economic and social environments in the North, South, East and West. These differences influence health and social policies in general and the strategies to prevent certain epidemics in particular. This becomes evident when we examine in detail the various prejudices, religious opinions and political motives regarding subjects like drug use and STDs. From a public health point of view it is imperative to develop a Pan-European strategy regarding infectious diseases, including a European approach to AIDS prevention.

On the several borders of the European Union, particularly along the borders shared with the newly independent states of Central and Eastern Europe, issues relating to HIV and other STD transmission are most visible and are a focus of public awareness and discussion. Especially the enormous increase in syphilis in Eastern Europe is often a topic at international meetings (for example, Swiss AIDS Federation, 1998). However, measures responding to the spread of STDs in these countries are quite rare, for several reasons. For example, most of the border regions tend to be rural, with larger cities and towns being the exception. Also, the health care infrastructure of each country is geared exclusively to the needs of their own population, the professional competency terminating at the border. In addition, services such as STD counselling and drug treatment – which are commonly available in Western European cities such as Berlin, Hamburg, Amsterdam, etc. – do not exist in these border regions. These are among the reasons why little has been undertaken to tackle the growth in drug use and prostitution.

We find in most border areas an established prostitution scene. Most active sex workers in Western European countries who are in touch with STD clinics and counselling centres are neither significantly affected by HIV nor by other sexually transmitted diseases (Heinz-Trossen, 1993). However, HIV infection continues to be an inherent risk in sex work, given the importance of sexual intercourse in the transmission of the disease. This is particularly true where the working environment of prostitutes is unsafe or highly competitive. The ability to make decisions regarding one's health and to take the necessary self-care measures may also be considerably impaired because of drug addiction, debt, poverty and external legal pressure (Steffan and Leopold, 1994).

Cross-national sex work is made possible by the increasing ease of international travel, the relatively short distances between countries, and the phenomenon of women from the East being able to undercut the going price for sexual services because of the vast differences in average income between their home countries and Western Europe. In general, border regions offer certain advantages for prostitution: clients and sex workers may remain anonymous (as they can cross the border to engage in prostitution as opposed to staying in their rural community) and differences between legal systems provide loopholes for prostitution.[1]

Since the unification of Germany sex work has changed due to an influx of women from neighbouring countries, particularly Poland, the Czech Republic, Slovakia, Bulgaria, and from the former Soviet Union (Russia, Ukraine and the Baltic States). Women from these countries can now return home more quickly than before, this increased mobility making typical health prevention work almost impossible.

Cross-border drug scenes have been identified so far in the regions between Poland and Germany, the Czech Republic and Germany, Italy and Slovenia, and Portugal and Spain. Commonly, such drugs as heroin, cocaine and special drugs like the so-called 'Polish soup' (an opiate in liquid form which is injected) are bought and sold, thus posing an additional threat for HIV transmission. A high prevalence of HIV within the respective drug using populations has been reported on the Polish-German border near Görlitz/Scorzelec and on the Portuguese-Spanish border around the Spanish town of Vigo (Steffan, Leopold *et al.*, 1997). In all these regions we see a connection between drug trafficking and prostitution because a growing number of young female addicts finance their use through sex work (Steffan, Leopold *et al.*, 1997).

The Umbrella Network

SPI-Research gGmbH has planned, implemented, supported, and evaluated a network of outreach projects called the Umbrella Network, focusing on HIV and STD prevention in border regions in Europe. This effort is supported by the European Commission (the funding and administrative body of the European Union); the Federal Ministry for Health in Germany; the German states of Bavaria, Saxony, Brandenburg and Mecklenburg-Western Pomerania; as well as by the EU countries of Greece, Austria, Finland, Italy, Spain and Portugal. In addition, funding is provided by the following countries: Switzerland, Estonia, Poland, the Czech Republic, Albania, Bulgaria and Slovenia.

The individual projects in the Umbrella Network have been working in various time frames, each project funded for a period of approximately three years. Up to this point thirteen pilot projects have been established in various border locations across Europe. Some of these projects have been in existence since the end of 1993.

The Network has the following goals:

- To analyse the risk potential of STD and HIV transmission in these regions.
- To disseminate prevention information regarding HIV and other STDs.
- To establish bilateral co-operation between the respective countries among the various institutions responsible for the target groups involved.
- To promote institutional assistance to target groups and, whenever possible, to develop new ways of delivering health care services.

To meet these goals, the Umbrella Network provides technical support and training, dissemination of lessons learned in the pilot programs, financial support in co-ordination with the European Commission, and the collection of data for the purpose of evaluation.

The general approach of all Umbrella Network projects is to establish bi-national, multilingual teams addressing health care and social needs of the respective populations on both sides of the border, setting up border crossing networks, offering counselling services, and participating in campaigns to overcome discrimination. The key approach adopted in this context has been outreach-based social work, which has made it possible to implement prevention strategies and to create access to the standard heath and social service agencies for the clientele in the target groups.

In general our working hypotheses is that isolated measures undertaken by a single state will not provide solutions to problems raised by cross-border sex work or drug dealing. What is required is bi-national, regional co-operative relationships between countries in order to offer the following services:

- Multilingual information and education.
- Ready access to condoms and lubricants.
- Improvement in the working conditions of prostitutes.
- Access to health care services including medical exams for (foreign) prostitutes.
- Involvement of sex workers in prevention work.
- Prevention campaigns addressing the clients of prostitutes.

It is very important that prevention not only include the distribution of condoms and syringes and testing people for HIV, but also that it be achieved through several additional measures:

- Providing information to the target group about HIV and other STDs.
- Influencing behaviour so as to promote more effective risk management among the target groups. By understanding the psychological factors and social circumstances influencing individuals' behaviour it is easier to find ways of helping them to adopt successful prevention strategies.
- Influencing the individual's environment. Living conditions can both facilitate and inhibit efforts to change behaviour. Therefore, the stabilisation of living conditions, particularly meeting basic needs, must be included in prevention work.

- Combating discrimination and criminalisation of the target groups. Marginalisation, discrimination and criminalisation make it difficult for affected individuals and groups to act in health-conscious ways.

HIV and STD prevention on the eastern border of Germany

Detailed information is currently available on prostitution and the drug trade in the border region of Poland and the German states of Mecklenburg-Western Pomerania and Brandenburg. There is also data for the states of Saxony and Bavaria regarding activity on the border of the Czech Republic as well as for Finland on the border of Estonia and Russia. Given the focus of this chapter, the following will describe the situation in the regions between Germany and Poland and Germany and the Czech Republic.

The six teams working since 1994 along the Polish/German and Czech/German borders have conducted approximately 50,000 units of counselling to prostitutes during more than 3,000 outreach shifts.[2] Outreach is conducted twice a week. Longer-term counselling relationships have been established with more than 4,000 prostitutes. Specifically-targeted HIV/AIDS prevention campaigns have been carried out periodically by all projects. Water-based lubricants are virtually unknown to many prostitutes. This is an important knowledge gap, given that oil-based products can lead to condom breakage. Promoting the proper use of lubricants is therefore an important task of the outreach teams.

The prostitutes' knowledge about STDs and HIV is generally quite poor at point of first contact with the teams. There is the additional problem of a constant fluctuation of about 30 per cent in the prostitute population, with new women being encountered during each outreach shift. The teams attempt to set up medical exams and diagnostic tests free of charge and anonymously, services which are not common in most of the border regions. Access to these forms of care are particularly important for prostitutes who are not from the host country because they usually have no health insurance and no residency permit.

All prostitutes who are in regular contact with the teams report attempting always to use condoms when having sex with clients. However, many women recount that clients often offer more money for unprotected sex and that it is difficult to refuse the added income when business is poor. An additional problem is that most women do not speak the language of their clients very well, requiring that methods of negotiation, other aspects of professional conduct, and self-defence techniques be taught in order to make consistent preventive behaviour possible.

In general, it can be said that the number of prostitutes in border regions, especially on the eastern border of the EU, is still rising. All projects working in these areas have also noted a dramatic increase in the potential for violence on the part of pimps and clients, whilst the trafficking of women is also on the increase. The number of women working voluntarily as prostitutes out of economic necessity is decreasing.

Evidently, in all project areas, the number of medical exams has risen as a result of the outreach work. The intensive contacts maintained with institutions in Poland and the Czech Republic as well as the continuous public relations work carried out by the projects and the SPI are also proving to be successful as measured by the following criteria:

1   Reaching the target group.
2   Inclusion of the target group within the prevention work.
3   Behaviour change and improved knowledge among those women with whom the projects have ongoing contact.
4   Establishing networks.
5   Lessening discrimination and prejudice on the part of organisations on both sides of the border.
6   Establishing relationships with medical providers.

Information gathered by the projects also indicates that prostitutes are migrating from Eastern Europe and that many of these women regularly move from country to country within the EU.

The Umbrella Network survey

Here we examine selected results of an ongoing survey that the Umbrella Network projects conduct during the course of their work. The data are from surveys in the border regions of Germany/Poland and Germany/Czech Republic which were collected during three waves of the survey: 1996, 1997–8, and 1998–9. The survey was administered to gather descriptive data about the population, with a focus on the social and health care situation of prostitutes working in these regions. The instrument is a questionnaire which was developed by the outreach workers based on conversations with women from the target group. The questionnaire is composed partially of standardised items concerning age, nationality, number of children, age of first sex work, reason for beginning sex work, experiences with pimps, experiences with violence, mobility, sexual practices, social situation, health, etc. The questions address twenty-three different dimensions.

The sample

To date a convenience sample of 388 prostitutes has been interviewed by the six projects in these border regions from 1996–9 (1996, n=160; 1997–8 n=114; 1998–9, n=114). All of the women participating in the research had been clients of the projects over a longer period of time; consequently, first-time contacts and women who were newcomers to the specific location or to prostitution were not included. The sample cannot claim to be representative for the population of women working as prostitutes in the border regions because we do not know how the subjects interviewed differ from the women refusing to provide information. Random, stratified, or purposeful sampling was not used as these methods would have disrupted the relationships established between the outreach workers and the prostitutes. The results do, however, depict important issues in the lives of women in these regions which have been observed over time by the outreach workers and SPI staff.

Results

Nationality

Most of the women interviewed in 1998–9 on the border of Germany/Poland and Germany/Czech Republic came from the Czech Republic (32 per cent), followed by the Ukraine (25 per cent), Poland (12 per cent), Slovakia (7.9 per cent), Russia (6 per cent), Bulgaria (5 per cent) and Belarus (4.5 per cent). A woman from South America and one from Thailand were encountered for the first time since the beginning of the survey. The composition of the sample according to nationality differs by location. For example, Czech women comprise the majority of subjects in the Czech Republic but are also found on the Polish border. Polish women, on the other hand, are found more often on the German side of the border (see below); whereas, on the Polish side one finds more women from the Ukraine and Belarus. The composition by nationality has also changed considerably since 1996. Czech women accounted for 40 per cent of the total in 1996, 37 per cent in 1997–8, and 32 per cent in 1998–9 indicating that their numbers have fallen considerably. A similar trend is evident for Bulgarian women who composed 14 per cent of the sample in 1996, dropping to 5 per cent in 1998–9. In contrast there has been an increase in the share of Ukrainian women from 6 per cent in 1996 to more than 14 per cent in 1997–8, with their proportion rising to 25 per cent in 1998–9. The last survey also included women from Lithuania and Romania (2 per cent in each case) for the first time. (See Figure 16.1.)

A comparison between the border regions of Germany/Poland and Germany/Czech Republic reveals that Polish women constitute a minority of the prostitutes in the Polish border region (12 per cent of subjects); whereas Czech women continue to be the largest national grouping along the Czech border (46.7 per cent). As both Polish and Czech women are allowed to travel to Germany without a visa, other factors must be playing a role. One explanation could be differing attitudes toward prostitution in the two countries. It has been our impression over time that the more strongly religious character of Polish society promotes a less permissive attitude toward prostitution, thus resulting in less women pursuing this source of income.

Age

The youngest person interviewed (1998–9) was 10 years old and the oldest was 55. The average age was 25 in 1998–9 (median 21). The age range has increased over time (1996: 16–46, 1997–8: 10–50), and the median age has fallen slightly

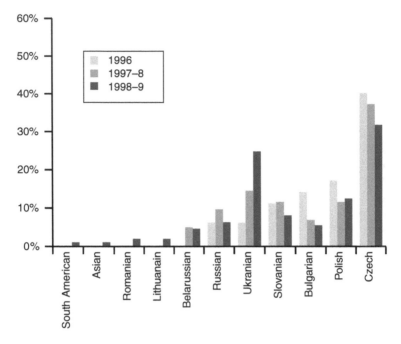

Figure 16.1 Nationality of the women in the survey

(23 in 1996; 22 in 1997–8; 21 in 1998–9). A growing number of children have been encountered in the course of the outreach work, particularly in Adorf/Cheb (Germany/Czech Republic). The KARO project in the region is co-operating with Czech institutions (with the support of the German state government of Saxony) in developing measures against child abuse.

Length of work

The women sampled had generally worked as prostitutes for six months to nine years. The average length of time for working as a prostitute was 3.2 years. This data may be skewed by the sampling procedure, given that only women known to the projects for a period of time were interviewed. In spite of this potential bias, less than one quarter of those interviewed had been working as prostitutes for one year or less. Lack of knowledge and an uncertainty when negotiating safer sex with clients has been observed by the outreach workers, particularly amongst this less experienced group.

Forced prostitution and pimping

The number of women claiming to have entered prostitution voluntarily has declined considerably. In 1998–9, 47 per cent of the women stated that this was the case, in contrast to 63 per cent in 1996. In 1998–9, more than half (53 per cent) of the women reported that the process of becoming a prostitute was accompanied by being forced or deceived into performing the work. The great majority of the women (99 per cent) in 1998–9 stated that they worked for pimps; whereas, in 1996 23 per cent of the women stated that they worked without a pimp.

Violence

On the whole, an increase in physical and sexual violence can be observed in the prostitution scene during the period the survey has been conducted. The interviews reveal an increase in violence against the women perpetrated by pimps: physical violence increased from 41 per cent (1996) to 58 per cent (1998–9) and sexual violence from 21 per cent (1996) to 30 per cent (1998–9). In 1997–8, 43 per cent of the women were subjected to violence by their clients, and 37 per cent stated that the police had also subjected them to physical violence.

This development may explain the continued feeling of helplessness and the increasing demand experienced by the respective regional infrastructures trying to assist the prostitutes. Apart from our projects, the police (during the occasional raid) are the only others from outside the prostitution scene who have contact with the women.

Health status

Data on the health status of the women were also gathered via the interview process. These data are self-reported and are not corroborated by clinical measures. Only one project is in a position to carry out medical examinations at present. All of the other projects work with STD counselling centres or clinics, and with physicians in private practice. The great number of cases of non-specific abdominal symptoms reported by the women (in 1996, 45 per cent of those interviewed claimed to suffer from such symptoms; this figure was 42 per cent in 1998–9) can be explained to some extent by a lack of knowledge concerning possible causes due to having no access to regular medical care. (See Figure 16.2.)

Of the prostitutes who had received medical exams, which has itself increased over time (1996: 32 per cent; 1997–8: 42 per cent; 1998–9: 56 per cent), 15.7 per cent (1996) stated that they had chlamydia (14 per cent in 1998–9), followed by syphilis (10.2 per cent in 1996 versus 13 per cent in 1998–9) and gonorrhoea (7.4 per cent in 1996 versus 6 per cent in 1998–9). Of those questioned, other conditions not directly related to sexually transmitted diseases were mentioned by 18.5 per cent in 1996 and by 17 per cent in 1998–9 (for example, colds, depression, allergies, skin diseases and alcoholism). All in all, the state of health of the women working as prostitutes in the border regions is still severely impaired as compared, for example, to prostitutes seeking services at STD counselling facilities in Germany in general (Heinz-Trossen, 1993).

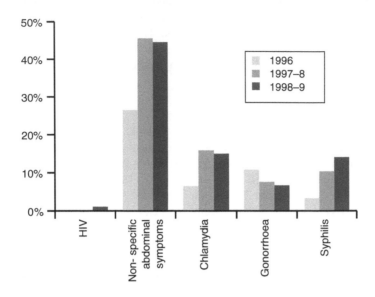

Figure 16.2 Self-reported STDs of the women in the survey

Conclusion

Our surveys of prostitutes within the border regions between German and Poland and Germany and the Czech Republic show a trend of the population becoming increasingly younger and therefore more inexperienced. There are also more women from other Eastern European countries – particularly the Ukraine, Belarus and the Baltic States – which has intensified the competition in an already competitive environment. This has resulted in a fall in prices for sex work, making it more possible for the customers of these women to impose unprotected sex. The readily apparent poverty of the women and pressure from pimps, combined with the women's inexperience and their isolation and language difficulties in a foreign country, also contribute to the prevalence of higher risk sexual practices. This is in contrast to the situation of 'professional' prostitutes in Germany.

It has been the experience of the Umbrella Network that co-ordinated health policy measures for the prevention of HIV and STDs in border-crossing prostitution and drug scenes are important. Lessons learned thus far include the following:

- With a prevalence of STDs rising as high as 30 per cent (the percentage of women with STDs examined in the project located in Domaslicze) border-crossing prostitution and drug scenes represent a particularly relevant target group for HIV and STD prevention.
- Outreach work greatly facilitates the establishment of contact with these target groups.

- Within the scope of the project work it was possible to obtain valuable information on the structures and characteristics of the various scenes. This knowledge is important for creating local infrastructures for providing prevention and care within a European framework.
- The scope of the outreach work performed for STD and HIV prevention, in accordance with the WHO Ottawa Charter and the tenets of structural prevention (see Etgeton, Chapter 7), aims to boost women's self-confidence in general as well as their consciousness of health issues. Stabilisation of their sense of efficacy fosters the development of new perspectives for independent living and helps them to overcome fear. It also creates a greater demand for support services, including assistance to leave prostitution work.
- Outreach workers are generally the only people to whom prostitutes in the border regions have any contact outside the prostitution scene. These staff are thus very important in organising more comprehensive assistance strategies.
- The problems arising in border-crossing prostitution cannot be solved at a national or bi-national level. In the near term, a political solution should be negotiated at the European level to make access to national health care services possible for immigrant populations working in border regions.

Notes

1 An example of how the differences in legal systems can promote the practice of cross-national prostitution can be found in the case of Switzerland and Sweden. Swiss men travel to Vorarlberg in Sweden where laws against hiring prostitutes are not as strictly enforced as in their own country.
2 The length of the units varies by region and counselling situation. For example, contacts on the street are generally briefer than those in clubs.

References

Gersch, C., Heckmann, W., Leopold, B. and Seyrer, Y. (1988) *Drogenabhängige Prostituierte und ihre Freier. SPI-Berlin, im Auftrag des Senators für Wissenschaft und Forschung, Berlin*, Berlin: SPI-Forschung.

Heinz-Trossen, A. (1993) *Prostitution und Gesundheitspolitik: Prostituiertenbetreuung als paedagogischer Auftrag des Gesetzgebers an die Gesundheitsaemter. Europaeische Hochschulschriften, Reihe 22, Soziologie; Bd. 239*, Frankfurt/Main: P. Lang.

Kleiber, D. and Velten, D. (1994) *Prostitutionskunden. Eine Untersuchung über soziale und psychologische Charakteristika weiblicher Prostituierter in den Zeiten von AIDS*, Baden-Baden: Nomos Verlagsgesellschaft.

Kleiber, D., Wilke, M., Soellner, R. and Velten, D. (1995): *AIDS, Sex und Tourismus. Ergebnisse einer Befragung deutscher Urlauber und Sextouristen*, Baden-Baden: Nomos Verlagsgesellschaft.

Leopold, B. and Steffan E. (1997) *EVA-Projekt. Evaluierung unterstützender Maßnahmen beim Ausstieg aus der Prostitution*, Berlin: SPI-Forschung.

Leopold, B., Steffan, E. *et al.* (eds) (1994) *Dokumentation zur sozialen und rechtlichen Situation von Prostituierten in Deutschland*, Stuttgart, Berlin, Cologne and Bonn: BMFJ.

SPI-forschung gGmbH (1998) *The Umbrella Network--A European Pilot Programme for HIV and STD Prevention in Border Regions*, Berlin: SPI-forschung gGmbH.

Steffan, E. and Leopold, B. (1994) 'Border crossing area prostitution and risk of HIV', in D. Friedrich and W. Heckmann (eds), *AIDS in Europe – The Behavioural Aspect*, Berlin: edition sigma, vol. 2: 207–13.

Steffan, E., Leopold, B. *et al.* (1997) *Abschlußbericht der wissenschaftlichen Begleitung des Modellprogramms 'Streetwork zur AIDS-Prävention im grenzüberschreitenden Raum'*, Bonn: Bundesministerium für Gesundheit.

Swiss AIDS Federation (1998) Second International Symposium on HIV Prevention: *Symposium Report*. Geneva: Swiss AIDS Federation.

Umbrella Network (1998) *Darstellung eines Europäischen Modellprogramms zur HIV/AIDS- und STD-Prävention im grenzüberschreitenden Raum*, Berlin: SPI-Forschung.

17 Innovation versus normalisation

The reaction of Germany's home care system to HIV and AIDS

Doris Schaeffer

Introduction

Hardly any other field of health care is under such great pressure to restructure and implement change as nursing in Germany is today. New social challenges have generated pressure to make innovations in many areas of nursing. This is due mainly to evolving structures for the elderly; a new panoply of diseases; the modifications, cutbacks and enhancements in the health care system; as well as a new legal climate. A slew of problems requiring solutions are beginning to be addressed – old problems which experts have warned about for decades. It is assumed that successful approaches are possible if given enough resolve, faith being placed in the ability of the system to make changes and innovations spontaneously. But this assumption has to be called into question, as the experience with AIDS has shown. The aim of this chapter is to present the positive and negative reactions of the home care nursing sector to HIV and AIDS in Germany and to ask what lessons we can take from this experience to be applied more generally to current issues in nursing.

In retrospect, AIDS can be understood as a pilot project in which the health care system's ability to make innovations was put to the test. With the unexpected emergence of this serious and often fatal disease, people in every area of health care – including home care services – were challenged to find new ways of working. It was necessary to perform a great number of services unrelated to any specific disease, services that are once again on the agenda. This includes home care care of the severely ill and making it possible for people to die humanely in their accustomed surroundings while including significant others in their care. Seen in this light, AIDS was, to a certain extent, the first test case. Did home care nursing pass the test?

AIDS meets home care in Germany

When a hitherto unknown contagious disease suddenly turned up about two decades ago in the form of AIDS, the pressure exerted on society soon became enormous. Although the belief that AIDS was an American phenomenon of little relevance to Germany prevailed initially at the political level (Frankenberg, 1994), this soon proved to be fallacious. The first cases of AIDS were reported in Germany in 1982: only one year later than in the US.

Although there were only fourteen cases that year, two years later there were already 320 and, in early 1990, 6,200 (Frankenberg, 1994: 138). A total of 17,995 cases of AIDS have been reported, and the number of confirmed positive HIV tests amounts to more than 130,000 (see Marcus, Chapter 3). In the course of the 1980s it soon became apparent that Germany also required an AIDS policy.

The strategy that gained acceptance after a brief and heated controversy did not follow the traditional model of epidemic control, but sought a new way of dealing with the social impact of the disease. Instead of relying on control and containment, it aimed for integration, with a patient-centred orientation being the guiding principle (for an account of the policy debate see Frankenberg and Hanebeck, Chapter 4). This meant that the ill were to receive care according to the specifics of their disease and their social situation. Furthermore, their quality of life and their autonomy were to be maximized in the time left to them; therefore, as much care as possible was to be provided on a home care basis. To implement this principle, the health care system needed to prove it was willing to make adjustments and innovations. Experience in the US had shown that, even in the case of such a severe disease as AIDS, hospitalisation was required only sporadically and care could be provided largely on a home care basis. It was, however, unclear how this could be done in Germany, given the following characteristics of the health care system:

- The dominance of the inpatient sector.
- An inadequate infrastructure for home care. For example, the expansion of home care providers did not begin until the end of the 1970s. As a consequence, some services required for home care were still lacking and others were unsatisfactorily organised. To the extent it was available, home care existed only as an adjunct service, even though it played a central role in the everyday life of certain patient groups (Garms-Homolová and Schaeffer, 1992).
- Deficient funding for home care, particularly for community nursing.
- Insufficient capacity in existing home-based services as well as a narrow focus on a specific clientele, namely older patients with chronic/degenerative diseases. Younger patients, particularly those from marginalised groups (for example, homosexuals and IV drug users), as well as patients with severe acute diseases still rarely receive home care (Schaeffer 1997, 1998; Ewers and Schaeffer, 1999).
- A narrow range of home care which does not provide all the services needed for the sick to remain at home. For example, in the mid-1980s the largest patient group using home-based services, the aged, were dying in hospitals (Novak, 1989). These were the years when AIDS patients were to be provided with the support needed in order to die humanely in their accustomed surroundings. This state of affairs can be attributed mainly to the characteristic tendency of the German health care system to hospitalise the sick, thus placing strict limits home care.

The pilot projects of the Federal Government

Clearly, it was necessary to increase both the quantity and quality of home care services. For this purpose special pilot projects in community nursing care were commissioned by the Federal Government in the second half of the 1980s.[1] This programme had the the following goals (see Wyns and Borchers, 1992; Schaeffer and Moers, 1995):

- To create an adequate infrastructure in community nursing and home care through the provision of additional personnel. All in all, 206 positions were created, being assigned to more than 35 locations throughout the entire country.
- To develop new home care models to address specifically the complex problems of the disease, including needs assessment and planning.
- To enable AIDS patients to receive care on a home care basis, even in the late stages of the disease, and to provide in-home palliative care.
- To test the feasibility of implementing new models within the existing structures of home care.
- To establish closely-knit networks of co-operation with other health providers in order to create the conditions necessary for patients to be able to remain at home and also to receive continuous and integrated care.

A study was commissioned by the Social Science Research Centre in Berlin (WZB) with the support of the Federal Ministry for Research and Technology (BMFT) and the Berlin Senate Office for Science and Research to investigate the care provided to AIDS patients in Germany. Within the context of this work, we investigated *inter alia* the extent to which the pilot projects have been successful in reaching the goals listed above. Here we will present the most important findings of this research.[2]

Sample

Given that the study was focused on services in Berlin, all home care organisations in that city participating in the pilot project were included. This comprised all the AIDS teams of the home care services managed by the Social Welfare Associations as well as private service providers who had AIDS patients in their care (see Wright, Chapter 2, for further information about the Social Welfare Associations). Data was collected from 1992–4. Each AIDS team was interviewed twice in order to observe how care is provided over time. The number of projects in Berlin was too small for making comparisons between groups and to provide enough data for each of the subject areas under study. For that reason, additional interviews were conducted in two other HIV epicentres, Munich and Frankfurt, which provided the additional data needed to ensure valid and generalisable findings. The total sample consisted of twenty-three interviews, eleven from AIDS teams in the Social Welfare Associations and nine within private home care agencies. Of the twenty-three interviews, seventeen were conducted in Berlin, with the rest being conducted in Frankfurt and Munich.

Method

Grounded Theory was the methodological basis for the study (Strauss, 1987; Glaser, 1978; Glaser and Strauss, 1962). Data collection proceeded, therefore, according to an inductive process, periods of interviewing alternating with periods of analysis in order to provide an ongoing process of contrasting case material. Data was collected through face-to-face interviews composed of open-ended questions, allowing interviewees ample opportunity to discuss their points-of-view while retaining the full narrative character of their responses.

Interview questions covered all areas of nursing care, with a particular focus on the attempts of the organisations to adapt care practices and structures to the needs of people with HIV/AIDS and to the challenges presented by HIV as a disease. Special attention was given to the ways in which co-ordinated and continuous care was being provided, given the tendency in the German health care system toward a lack of service integration. Concretely, the interview covered the specific aspects of AIDS patient care (outpatient and inpatient medical and home care, psychosocial services, etc.), posing questions concerning the nursing and other care needs of AIDS patients, concepts for AIDS nursing care, the organisation of the work, internal and external co-operation and communication, co-operation with other AIDS providers, interactions with patients and their significant others, and difficulties encountered in the daily work.

The findings of the study will be summarised here by presenting three typical home care nursing responses to HIV/AIDS in Germany as demonstrated by the organisations interviewed.

Normalisation as leitmotif

The first model to be mentioned here was demonstrated by one of the four independent Social Welfare Associations who are active on a nationwide basis and who are responsible for most home care services.

The Berlin regional office of this Association was included in the study. This office is responsible for twelve nursing agencies which received four nursing positions and one social worker for the care of AIDS patients within the context of the aforementioned pilot program. The new staff were not to assume 'the role of a 'hands-on' AIDS-nurse' (Wanjura, 1988: 776). The patients were instead supposed to be directly placed with the nursing agencies according to the usual method. The AIDS team, composed of the newly-hired nurses and the social worker, was to collaborate closely with these agencies, providing them with consultation so as to help them develop appropriate approaches to nursing for AIDS patients. Thus, the AIDS team was primarily supposed to have a training role, preparing the existing nursing staff of the twelve agencies for the new group of patients by way of conveying concrete know-how.

This model of care is based on two primary assumptions:

- The primary challenge of HIV/AIDS was viewed by the Social Welfare Association as being one of adaptation on the part of staff. Thus, consultation between AIDS team and other nursing providers was the focus.
- AIDS patients were to be integrated into the regular care system, bringing about a normalisation of their situation, thus avoiding discrimination and marginalisation.

The goal of integrating AIDS patients into the larger system is laudable; however, the typical services available were not up to the task. Briefly, typical care consists of housekeeping, nursing care, psychosocial support from a social worker, and – at least theoretically – all other tasks arising in connection with AIDS. In everyday practice, however, the range of services is far narrower. The following are seldom available: nursing for the seriously ill; IV therapy; support for family members; hospice care; psychosocial support; twenty-four-hour nursing care; and crisis intervention services. The latter are disruptive to the organisational and financial structures found in most nursing agencies and, in certain cases, are severely limited legally (for example, IV therapy).[3]

It is therefore no wonder that the course taken by this model – like that of many others, as well – is one of failure characterised by mutually intensifying defensive reactions. The AIDS team did not succeed in building functional collaborative structures with other members of the nursing staff. Regardless of the strategy chosen, the team met with resistance on the part of the nurses, who wanted nothing to do with AIDS and AIDS patients, effectively closing the door to the AIDS team.

The failure of this model has grave consequences for AIDS patients. To this day, nurses in these agencies often react with avoidance and selectivity when dealing with problems related to this patient group. They provide AIDS patients with only sporadic care and only when the patients' needs are compatible with the current range of available services, that is, when no IV therapy is required, no extensive psychosocial care is needed, and no other tasks arise which go beyond usual care. A continuity of care is also not available because of the lacking collaboration and co-ordination with other institutions involved in providing services for AIDS patients. If AIDS patients are provided with care, this is usually done only at an early stage of the disease. In the later stages, when the need for nursing care intensifies and is no longer compatible with the usual tasks performed, patients suddenly find themselves seeking help elsewhere (most typically at nursing agencies specialising in AIDS care, where available, or in hospitals). This help-seeking behaviour of patients due to inadequacies in home care nursing have been confirmed in another study in progress which documents care paths taken by AIDS patients (Schaeffer, Moers and Rosenbrock, 1992).

The experience gathered in implementing a normalisation approach shows in exemplary fashion that the adjustment to HIV and AIDS on the part of the typical nursing providers has been highly deficient. This is all the more lamentable, since these services account for the majority of nursing care in Germany's home care sector. The reasons for the failure are several.

First, it should be noted that the AIDS team – like many other staff providing nursing care (Schaeffer and Moers, 1995; Schaeffer, 1991) – received no assistance whatsoever from the Social Welfare Association; that is, the parent organisation of the nursing providers. The Association may have been prepared to avail itself of the financial opportunities made possible through AIDS work, but it would not commit itself to developing appropriate care. From the very beginning, the team received no assistance in performing its tasks nor was it provided with the necessary expertise and independence in order to develop their role. There was also no response from the Association when the team met with difficulties in implementing the proposed changes. Such deficits are one of the primary reasons for the poor success achieved with the adaptation measures.

Second, the Social Welfare Association's concept proved not to be viable. The normalisation strategy was unable to cope with the problems that had arisen. For one, the strategy prevented the special nursing needs of this patient group from being identified, and it impeded the development of appropriate nursing concepts. In addition, it soon became clear that the provision of services on a largely home care basis is not possible for the seriously ill without expanding the limited range of services available from the nursing agencies, which would mean changing the way they operate. The fact that this did not happen led, in effect, to the opposite of what the pilot project was trying to achieve. That is, the patients were expected to adjust to the needs of the service provider rather than the other way around.

Third, implementing the collaboration with the AIDS team proved to be impossible. Fears of infection and an aversion to people with AIDS played an important role. At the same time, there were strategic reasons for the opposition. The nursing staff resisted taking on more work resulting from the growing number of tasks. This work was incompatible with the structures of the usual community nursing care and thus had to be performed as special services or as services requiring extra personnel. Furthermore, staff feared that these new services would have to be made available in the future to other groups of patients, as well. This premonition has proved to be correct. In Germany, there is much current discussion concerning a more radical application of home care in place of inpatient care. One reason is that caring for AIDS patients has shown that the severely ill can be provided nursing on a home care basis. Seen in this light, the refusal of nursing staff to co-operate points out the problematic situation of community nursing care in Germany and illustrates that staff cannot be expected to change their behaviour without simultaneous structural changes in community nursing itself.

Fourth, regarding the AIDS team, it is also necessary to mention the lack of fit between the job descriptions and staff qualifications. The duties of the AIDS team belong to the realm of public health nursing and require various competencies (for example, teaching, programme planning and implementation, and the development of co-ordinating structures). These activities have little in common with the skills imparted by nursing education in Germany which was conceived of as three years of practical occupational training emphasizing hands-on care-giving. In countries with an academic tradition of nursing (for example, the US), advanced training, nursing education, structural changes, theoretical work, etc. are the domain of the academically educated nurses (see Schaeffer, 1995b). This problem of fit and qualification has contributed decisively to the failure of the normalisation model, reflected in the inadequate manner in which the team members implemented their goals, their inability to conceptualise their tasks appropriately, their development of ineffective procedures for the given goal and task, and the personalising of conflicts.

Innovation as a leitmotif

The second example is a specialised AIDS nursing agency which arose from the gay movement as a grass-roots project. This provider has succeeded in reacting to the AIDS crisis in an innovative fashion. From the beginning, the focus was on direct care of AIDS patients, with the agency defining itself to be a 'nursing service for the severely ill' (Weber, 1992). From the conceptual, practical and organisational point of view, the agency was based on the principle of patient-oriented care. Services supported for a period of four years under the federal pilot project programme resulted in hiring four nurses and one social worker. Today it employs a staff of thirty-three, mainly nurses and housekeepers, but also a social worker, two psychologists, and a director entrusted with administrative tasks and other management functions. As with the nursing agencies in Berlin, the service profile includes housekeeping, nursing care and social work. In addition, hospice care, psychosocial support, psychological service, and work with family members are offered. The range of tasks and their definitions are much broader than the services found under regular nursing care. Intensive home care, the performance of IV therapy, and twenty-four-hour nursing as well as palliative services are viewed as matters of course. The IV therapy was performed in such a way as to go around the regulations which prohibit this service on a home care basis. The concept envisages the following:

- To employ nursing care as early as possible so that prevention-oriented nursing care can be provided.
- To prioritise the patients' needs over organisational imperatives. Nursing care is structured in accordance with the clients' way of life, the nurse visiting at the convenience of the patient.
- To operate according to specific standards of practice, including care planning and evaluation. This is important, given that these principles have only begun to be instituted on a broad basis in Germany in the last few years.
- To ensure the patient's personal autonomy. He or she is included in all planning and decision-making; nursing is understood as a process of

negotiation. The innovation of this concept becomes clear when compared to the hierarchically structured German health care system. In this respect, too, AIDS acquired the function of a catalyst, and democratisation measures were initiated in many areas (Schaeffer, Moers and Rosenbrock, 1992).

- To implement nursing practices which recognise both the social and psychological well-being of patients. Social and psychological support is the task not only of the nursing staff but also of the social worker and the two psychologists employed specifically for this purpose. The personnel render competent help in psychological crises and when illness-related events have to be addressed.

- To view the patient as part of his or her social environment, including family members as constitutive elements in the care, and not focusing exclusively on the individual patient. Family members are supported in performing care-related tasks. They are also assisted in coping with the changes in their own lives brought about by the disease. This task, most commonly referred to in English as 'caring for the caregivers', is just now beginning to take hold, thanks to the Long-Term Care Insurance Act (see 'social insurances' in Wright, Chapter 2).

- To provide a continuity of care, for example, by visiting patients during temporary stays in the hospital and by bridging gaps in care when patients move from inpatient to home care.

- To continue providing care during periods of decline and during dying, making it possible for patients to stay in familiar surroundings as opposed to being referred to the hospital.

- To prioritise the organisation of care and the coordination of services while advocating for the patients' needs.

The agency also functions as a primary care system for the patient, providing a continuity of personnel. In standard nursing care in Germany, the rotation principle is followed, that is, care is provided by the particular personnel assigned at any given shift. Furthermore, there are regular weekly case conferences which all staff members providing care attend. Here the problems of individual patients are discussed, the services of the participating providers are co-ordinated, and service-related issues are resolved. These structures may not seem new or innovative, but up until recently it was not customary in Germany for home nursing providers to hold case conferences; now such meetings are required by law. The guiding principle of the agency is the idea of teamwork; that is, participation of all staff, regardless of professional qualification. Also, continuing education and advanced training are a standard, another feature which is not customary in German nursing practice.

Furthermore, to ensure integrated home care, a dense network of collaboration was created including AIDS specialists and other providers required for comprehensive patient care (other medical practices, hospitals, physical therapists, occupational therapists, psychosocial services, self-help groups, churches, funeral homes, health insurance companies, policy makers, etc.) This is also remarkable since it can only be done with a relatively large amount of co-ordinated effort and time, given the splintered nature and organisational separatism of the services involved in home care. Since such work cannot be billed, formal networking is usually neglected in nursing. Many new forms of co-operation with medical institutions have been tried which can serve as models for home care more generally (also see Schaeffer and Moers, 1995).

All of these innovations witness to the tremendous pioneering work which has been achieved by this agency. Some of the innovations have the character of overdue steps toward modernisation, others go even further. Many of the innovations are relevant for the care provided to other patients, not just people with AIDS, underlining the value of the experience gained here. Nevertheless, this model, too, has a number of weaknesses.

The limited capacity must be mentioned first and foremost. At an average of fifteen per project, the number of patients is relatively small. There are signs of imminent overloading, especially when palliative care is required simultaneously for a number of patients.

Many conceptual elements were formulated haphazardly and now require systematisation. That is not surprising since many different tasks had to be performed at the same time: development work, the creation of co-operative structures and networks, conceptualisation of needs and methods, and the provision of practical nursing. The profusion of tasks means that adjustments to changes in the progress of the disease and, in particular to AIDS becoming increasingly chronic in nature, are delayed and sometimes insufficient. Moreover, the multiple activities tend to place an excessive strain on staff, with burn-out being a constant issue.

In many cases, such innovative nursing agencies had to be reorganised. Their self-help character and the aim of providing professional nursing care were constantly interfering with each other. Reorganisation measures were usually linked to considerable personnel turnover, sometimes threatening the livelihood of the agencies. These and other instability phenomena can often be seen in the case of grass-roots enterprises. This has consequences for the patient in that he or she cannot be sure of finding a consistent range of services.

In everyday practice, the innovative agencies are constantly confronted with structural deficits, and above all, funding problems. This poses an ever lurking threat to their existence, tying up a great deal of resources which could be invested in other activities.

Improvement of image as leitmotif

In contrast to providers under the auspice of social service organisations, private agencies are organised as commercial enterprises. They have reacted more flexibly than the former (the first example given), but not with nearly as many innovations as the agencies specialised in AIDS care (the second example). In interest of space, the work of the private agencies will only be described here briefly.

Commercial nursing providers have existed in Germany since the mid-1980s and are presently expanding very rapidly. For many of them, AIDS proved to be an unforeseen opportunity to gain recognition, for they previously had a relatively poor public image. Everywhere they were stymied with the reputation of 'creaming', that is, selecting only easy-care and fully reimbursable cases, while leaving other patients to the voluntary services. Their reaction to HIV and AIDS proved this reputation to be unjustified. When it was apparent that the non-commercial nursing providers were afraid to deal with the disease thus avoiding AIDS patients, the private nursing agencies took up the challenge. In a short period of time, many of these providers – especially in cities of high HIV prevalence – adapted their service profile to the needs of the new patient group, qualified their nursing staff, and followed several AIDS patients on a continual basis. They have thus shown that AIDS care is commercially feasible. Certain reservations must, however, be mentioned.

In most cases, the structure of services was not significantly modified, the expansion of the service profile limited to nursing services directly tied to the physician's care. Several private nursing agencies hired a physician so as to legally safeguard the range of services they were able to offer. Although a sign of flexibility, this approach is contradictory from a policy point of view, in that the services rendered by the nursing staff are thus subjected to increasing physician control as opposed to providing more professional independence for nursing practice.

The large number of tasks required in the caring for AIDS patients usually have to be performed by the nursing staff as special services, and thus depend on the individual nurses' helpfulness and their capacity to respond.

As a rule, the private nursing providers do not have any psychologists or social workers on staff because there is no way to bill health insurance companies for their services. Housekeepers are also not usually on staff for the same reason. Those providers who have hired social workers tend to view assistance in the form of counselling on personal issues and help with concrete daily tasks as a waste of time. The focus is on producing visible results; for example, by arranging other services, clarifying financial questions, and organising service delivery to be more efficient. As for housekeeping chores, commercial cleaning firms are contracted to provide service to patients. Although this seems on the surface to be a reasonable and practical solution, the outsourcing of this service is not keeping with the principles of nursing which call for integrated care, as opposed to segmenting services into discrete tasks performed by different providers.

Collaborative structures exist primarily with medical providers; formal collaboration with social service agencies, self-help groups, psychotherapists, etc. is virtually non-existent.

In short, the drawback of the private nursing agencies is the limited range of services. If the need for care – particularly social and emotional support – increases, the services provided by the private agencies is often unsatisfactory. Patients experiencing complex social problems (for example, drug addiction, homelessness, etc.) are not accepted into care by these providers, given their limitations.

Summary and discussion

In retrospect, AIDS has created a quasi-experimental situation in which the health care system's flexibility and adaptability have been put to the test. The nursing care providers in Germany have just barely passed. A first attempt was made to make home nursing services available to the severely ill and to provide palliative care, thus tackling major shortcomings in Germany's health care system. However, the success of these efforts was limited. Once AIDS patients need home care, they cannot be certain of the type and range of services they will receive. Especially in the late stages of the disease and when the patient is dying, it is often impossible to maintain care primarily at home. Now in the second decade of HIV/AIDS, the sick are still confronted with avoidance and even incompetence, especially in non-specialised facilities providing general medical care. It was mainly the specialised nursing providers who reacted flexibly and innovatively to the AIDS crisis, followed by the private commercial providers. The specialised agencies care for most of the AIDS patients in Germany, being the first to be contacted by patients. Whether the available capacity can meet the demand is still a question, given that many specialized providers are hopelessly overburdened with the changing demands brought on them by AIDS becoming a more chronic illness and by their own financial difficulties. This rather negative conclusion is surprising, in view of the considerable funds made available in Germany in order to adapt home care to HIV and AIDS. The adjustment by outpatient nursing to AIDS, on the whole, has been less satisfactory and less innovative than other areas of the health care system. There are many reasons for this.

We conclude by summarising here the main barriers to innovation in nursing regarding AIDS care:

1   The reaction of the home care providers was characterised by a view of AIDS as being an exceptional disease (Schaeffer, 1993b). While the grass-roots agencies viewed the exceptional nature of AIDS as an interesting challenge, the regular health care system reacted to it with aversion. This is understandable to the extent that the home care services had not been confronted with infectious diseases of this magnitude for some time. Nevertheless, the consequence of this reaction was the inability to see the common problems between AIDS care and the care of people with other diseases, and the tendency to overlook the opportunity provided by AIDS to address important shortcomings of home care as a whole.

2   The diversity and volatility of the problems encountered in the practice of home care was underestimated at the political level. A continuous growth in new tasks has overburdened home-based services since the major impetus in the 1980s to develop home nursing care (Garms-Homolovà and Schaeffer, 1992). Lack of capacity and the narrow limits on the range of home-care activity result in overload and its accompanying organisational and personnel problems. Many providers thus feel unable to cope with unfamiliar demands, new groups of patients, and the additional tasks

required by AIDS. This explains why the readiness to adapt to the disease on a committed and active basis has remained relatively limited.

3   There has been an arrested development of Germany's nursing system, which makes itself felt in AIDS care. For some time now there has been a general consensus that nursing has been unable to keep up with the structural transformations in society, thus not in a position to meet the growing demands placed on services. In spite of this observation, change has failed to take place, until recently. Currently, the education of nurses is being reorganised, raising the level of qualification and expanding nursing practice beyond traditional areas of activity. This very late development, as compared to other countries, has not yet had any repercussions on everyday nursing. For the majority of nurses currently in practice, further training is only available in a fragmentary fashion, not adequately addressing the demands of their changing practice. This is especially true for home care, as home and community nursing are hardly taken into account in the education currently provided. Excessive demands, quality issues and opposition to new standards are the result. If the nursing system does not try to overcome this developmental shortcoming, it will hardly be in a position to meet new social demands and the need for change in the future.

4   Finally, experience shows what the consequences are when the importance of implementation and innovation management are underestimated. Although available studies keep pointing to the resistance of Germany's health care system to reform (for example, Rosewitz and Webber, 1990), politicians continue to have faith in the ability of the system to spontaneously adapt. This is a fallacy, as the experience gained in the area of AIDS once again confirms (see also Schaeffer and Moers, 1992; Schaeffer, 1993a). Lasting, realistic changes in the customary practice of nursing require vigilance and guidance if fatigue, gaffes and diversions are to be avoided. Not only the experience with AIDS but also the history of nursing shows that attempts at change and innovation are frequently doomed to failure. Therefore careful long-term planning is needed to avoid implementation obstacles and defensive reactions. Seen in this light, AIDS was an instructive pilot project which has been important, if only to draw attention to the existing deficits in nursing which have been in need of reform for some time.

Notes

1   The project began in 1987 and lasted four years. (See Wyns and Borchers, 1992.) Part of the Federal Goverment's Emergency Program to Fight AIDS called for a total of seven pilot projects. (See Schaeffer and Moers, 1995.)

2   See Schaeffer and Moers (1992, 1995) and Schaeffer (1995a, 1995b, 1996, 1997) for more detailed reports of the study's results.

3   Home nursing services in Germany do not provide for any differentiation of tasks or for vertical and horizontal division of labour. The nursing staff are generalists who

perform every required task, functioning essentially as skilled labourers. Being viewed as labourers and not as professionals also explains why the definition of tasks which can be performed is relatively narrow.

4   IV therapy is still only performed on an inpatient basis.

References

Ewers, M. and Schaeffer, D. (1999) *Herausforderungen für die ambulante Pflege Schwerstkranker. Eine Situationsanalyse nach Einführung der Pflegeversicherung. Veröffentlichungsreihe des Instituts für Pflegewissenschaft*, Bielefeld: Institut für Pflegewissenschaft: 99–107.

Frankenberg, G. (1994) 'Deutschland: Der verlegene Triumph des Pragmatismus', in D. Kirp and R. Bayer (eds), *Strategien gegen AIDS. Ein internationaler Politikvergleich. Ergebnisse sozialwissenschaftlicher AIDS-Forschung* vol. 14, Berlin: edition sigma: 134–72.

Garms-Homolová, V. and Schaeffer, D. (1992) *Versorgung alter Menschen. Sozialstationen zwischen wachsendem Bedarf und Restriktionen*. Freiburg: Lambertus.

Glaser, B. (1978) *Theoretical Sensitivity – Advances in the Methodology of Grounded Theory*, Mill Valley, Los Angeles: Sociology Press.

Glaser, B. and Strauss, A. (1962) *The Discovery of Grounded Theory: Strategies for Qualitative Research*, New York: Aldine.

Hamouda, O. *et al.* (1994) *AIDS/HIV 1993. Bericht zur epidemiologischen Situation in der Bundesrepublik Deutschland zum 31.12.1993*, Berlin: AIDS-Zentrum im Bundesgesundheitsamt.

Moers, M. and Schaeffer, D. (1992) 'Die Bedeutung niedergelassener Aerzte fuer die Herstellung von Versorgungsskontinuitaet bei Patienten mit HIV-Symptomen', in D. Schaeffer, M. Moers and R. Rosenbrock (eds), *AIDS-Krankenversorgung,* Berlin: edition sigma: 133–60.

—— (1993) *AIDS-Krankenversorgung in San Francisco. Innovative Versorgungsstrategien und Betreuungsmodelle. Paper der Forschungs-gruppe Gesundheitsrisiken und Praeventionspolitik,* Berlin: Wissenschaftszentrum Berlin fuer Sozialforschung: 93–203.

Novak, P. (1989) 'Grenzprobleme der Medizin', in F. Wagner (ed.), *Medizin. Momente der Veränderung*, Berlin, Heidelberg and New York: Springer: 43–63.

Rosewitz, B. and Webber, D. (1990) *Reformversuche und Reformblockaden im deutschen Gesundheitswesen*, Frankfurt/Main and New York: Campus.

Schaeffer, D. (1991) 'Probleme bei der Implementation neuer Versorgungsprogramme fuer Patienten mit HIV-Symptomen', *Neue Praxis* 5(6): 392–406.

—— (1993a) 'Integration von ambulanter und stationaerer Versorgung', in B. Badura, G. Feuerstein and T. Schott (eds), *System Krankenhaus*, Munich: Juventa: 270–91.

—— (1993b) 'Patientenorientierung und Gesundheitsfoerderung im Krankenhaus. Erfordernisse der Organisations- und Strukturentwicklung', in J. M. Pelikan, H. Demmer and K. Hurrelmann (eds), *Gesundheitsfoerderung durch Organisationsentwicklung. Konzepte, Strategien und Projekte fuer Betriebe, Krankenhaeuser und Schulen*, Munich: Juventa: 267–84.

—— (1994) 'Wissenstransfer im Gesundheitswesen. Analyse eines in der AIDS-Krankenversorgung erprobten Modells', *Neue Praxis, Zeitschrift fuer Sozialarbeit, Sozialpaedagogik und Sozialpolitik* 24(2): 154–67.

—— (1995a) Patientenorientierte Krankenversorgung: Aids als Herausforderung. *Zeitschrift für Gesundheitswissenschaften* 3(4): 332–48.

206   *D. Schaeffer*

—— (1995b) 'Pflegestudiengänge in den USA. Lernen für die Entwicklung im deutschsprachigen Raum', in A. Heller, D. Schaeffer and E. Seidl (eds), *Akademisierung von Pflege und Public Health*, Vienna, Munich and Bern: Wilhelm Maudrich: 127–48.

—— (1996) *Innovationsprozesse in der ambulanten Pflege. Aids als Pilotprojekt* 9(2): 140–9.

—— (1997) *Patientenorientierte ambulante Pflege Schwerkranker. Erfordnernisse der Konzept- und Wissenschaftsentwicklung. Zeitschrift für Gesundheitswissenschaften* 5(2): 85–97.

—— (1998) 'Die Versorgung von akut kranken Menschen durch integrierte ambulante Versorgungsverbünde in Deutschland', in J. M. Pelikan, A. Stacher, A. Grundböck and K. Krajic (eds), *Virtuelles Krankenhaus zuhause – Entwicklung und Qualität von ganzheitlicher Hauskrankenpflege*, Vienna: Faculta Universtätsverlag: 50–6.

Schaeffer, D. and Moers, M. (1992) 'Professionelle Versorgung von HIV- und AIDS-Patienten. Zwischenbericht des Projekts "Versorgung und Betreuung von Patienten mit HIV-Symptomen. Praeventive Potentiale kurativer Institutionen"', *Paper der Forschungsgruppe Gesundheitsrisiken und Praeventionspolitik*, Berlin: Wissenschaftszentrum Berlin fuer Sozialforschung: 92–208.

—— (1993) 'Professionell gebahnte Versorgungspfade und ihre Konsequenzen fuer die Patienten. Ergebnisse einer strukturanalytischen Untersuchung der AIDS-Krankenversorgung', in C. Lange (ed.), *AIDS – eine Forschungsbilanz*. Berlin: edition sigma: 59–74.

—— (1994) 'Praeventive Potentiale kurativer Institutionen – Praevention als Aufgabe ambulanter Pflege', in R. Rosenbrock, H. Kuehn and B. Koehler (eds), *Praeventionspolitik. Gesellschaftliche Strategien der Gesundheits-sicherung*, Berlin: edition sigma: 384–407.

—— (1995) 'Ambulante Pflege von HIV- und AIDS-Patienten', *Paper der AG Public Health*, Berlin: Wissenschaftszentrum Berlin fuer Sozial-forschung: 95–201.

Schaeffer, D., Moers, M. and Rosenbrock, R. (eds) (1992) *AIDS-Krankenversorgung*, Berlin: edition sigma.

—— (1992) 'AIDS-Krankenversorgung zwischen Modellstatus und Übergang in die Regelversorgung', in D. Schaeffer, M. Moers, and R. Rosenbrock (eds), *AIDS-Krankenversorgung*, Berlin: edition sigma: 11–25.

—— (eds) (1994) *Public Health und Pflege. Zwei neue gesundheitswissenschaftliche Disziplinen*, Berlin: edition sigma.

Strauss, A. (1987) *Qualitative Analysis for Social Scientists,* New York: Cambridge University Press.

Wanjura, M. (1988) *Ambulante Versorgung von AIDS-Patienten Deutsche Kranken-pflegezeitschrift,* 10: 754–6.

Weber, A. (1992) 'Grenzerfahrungen bei der ambulanten Pflege von Menschen mit HIV und AIDS', in D. Schaeffer, M. Moers and R. Rosenbrock (eds), *AIDS-Kranken-versorgung*, Berlin: edition sigma: 222–50.

Wyns, B. and Borchers, A. (1992) 'Moeglichkeiten und Grenzen der Versorgung HIV-Infizierter und AIDS-Kranker durch ambulante Pflegedienste und Sozialstationen', in D. Schaeffer, M. Moers and R. Rosenbrock (eds), *AIDS-Krankenversorgung*, Berlin: edition sigma: 197–221.

18 Defining the AIDS Survivor Syndrome and testing for symptoms in an exploratory study of gay German men

Michael T. Wright

Introduction

Since the beginning of the AIDS epidemic the group most directly affected by the disease in Germany has been gay men. Infection rates among this group well exceed those of the general population (Dannecker, 1990; Bochow, 1994; Marcus, Chapter 3) with the result that AIDS has become part of the everyday reality for many members of this community. Even for men who have not tested seropositive, the disease asserts its presence in the lives of friends and acquaintances and as a potential threat when having sex with other men.

This epidemiological phenomenon is compounded by the ongoing discrimination and marginalisation experienced by gay men in Germany (Bochow, 1993). Already burdened by the consequences of cultural homophobia, this subgroup has had to confront a serious and often fatal disease. The effect on gay men as a result of living through the epidemic is not clear. Martin Dannecker (1990) has suggested the existence of AIDS-related trauma reactions at both the collective and personal levels among gay men in Germany. Within this study, an attempt was made to identify trauma reactions in the form of an hypothesized AIDS Survivor Syndrome, this construct based on the extensive literature concerning other survivor syndromes. Exploratory interviews were conducted within a sample of gay German men to investigate under what circumstances such a syndrome may exist.

The Survivor Syndrome

The first description of a survival syndrome is found in the work of William G. Niederland, who in 1968 used the term to label the reactions of survivors from Nazi concentration camps. Although no conclusive definition of the syndrome exists in the literature, there is a constellation of signs and symptoms most often associated with this phenomenon: persistent arousal with an exaggerated startle response; avoidance of memories of the traumatic events; inner tension; ruminating; marked moodiness or irritability; emotional numbness; lack of initiative; apathetic withdrawing; restlessness; difficulties concentrating; lack of productivity; inability to find enjoyment and pleasure in life; meaninglessness in life as whole; nightmares or intrusive memories; low self-esteem; social isolation with a suspicion of others' motives; psychosomatic disturbances; and 'survival guilt' (Krystal and Niederland, 1968; Peters, 1989; Marcus and Rosenberg, 1988; Steinberg, 1989; Goderez, 1987; Jucovy, 1991; Eckstaedt, 1988). Krystal and Niederland (1968) felt that the so-called 'survival guilt' was the primary element of the syndrome, defining it as the feeling: 'Why me? Why did I survive when all of the others died? I should have died as well.'

Since the work of Niederland the term survival syndrome has been adopted by a range of authors to describe the reactions of people who survived other types of traumatic events, everything from war (Goderez, 1987; Herbst, 1992) and earthquakes to man-made disasters (Giel, 1991). Survivor syndrome theory is applied predominantly to situations in which a definable group of people is subjected to a catastrophic, life-threatening event. The literature, therefore, depicts the syndrome as being comprised of both individual and collective elements. The question in this study was whether the term can also be used to describe the lives of gay men in Germany living in the time of AIDS.

AIDS and the gay community

There is evidence in the literature that AIDS does, in fact, constitute a catastrophic event of the proportions to produce traumatic reactions as defined by a survivor syndrome.

Several American authors call attention to 'disenfranchised grief' among gay men. That is, given society's homophobia, men who lose friends and loved ones to AIDS do not have adequate opportunity to mourn their deaths (Sklar, 1991; Doka, 1989; Pine, 1989; Fuller et al., 1989; Dick, 1989; Hays et al., 1990). There is also the potential loss in terms of gay identity, given that AIDS has ushered in a fear and anxiety regarding sex which is anathema to the early gay movement (Schwartzberg, 1992; Klein and Fletcher, 1986; Dannecker, 1990; Hays et al., 1990). Psychotherapists working with gay men who have lost significant others to AIDS also report such problems as fear of death, phobic reactions to sexuality, avoidance of other gay men, psychosomatic and even psychotic reactions (Barrows and Halgin, 1988; Vogel, 1994; Odets, 1995). Other authors – from the US, Germany and Australia – attest to a fearful avoidance of sexual activity (Davidson, 1991; Viney et al., 1991; Odets, 1995; Dannecker, 1990). And, there are also reports from the US and Germany of guilt among gay men which resembles the survivor guilt first described by Niederland (Hakert, 1994; Vogel, 1994; Odets, 1995; Deutsche AIDS-Hilfe, 1993).

Two studies, conducted in Sydney (Viney et al., 1991) and New York (Martin, 1988; Martin and Dean, 1993; Martin et al., 1989; Lennon et al., 1990) provide empirical evidence to support the existence of such a phenomenon among gay men, documenting various negative psychological reactions to the AIDS epidemic. The New York study offers particularly compelling data, given the longitudinal design, the relatively large number of participants, and the nature of the instrument, which was developed over time and subjected to various statistical and field tests.

Based on the existing literature, the AIDS Survivor Syndrome (ASS) was defined for the purposes of this investigation as follows:

- Post Traumatic Stress Disorder symptoms directly related to experiences with HIV/AIDS.
- Complicated grief reactions to the death of significant others due to AIDS.
- Survival guilt.
- A heightened fear of death, fear of discrimination, and fear of one's own sexuality and of sexual contact with other men.
- High levels of internalised homophobia.
- Sexual disturbance associated with sexual dissatisfaction, fear, guilt, and sexual acting out.
- A tendency to take more risk of becoming infected with HIV.
- Social isolation.
- A lack of interest in talking about the traumatic experiences due to AIDS, even in the context of close relationships.

Also, based on the literature, one would expect to see more symptoms among those men who have had intimate contact with those who have died, those who are HIV positive, those isolated from others in the same situation, those without long-term coping strategies, and those who do not have clear limits in their life concerning the issue of HIV/AIDS.

Sample

The sample consisted of sixty-five gay-identified men from throughout Germany. A convenience sampling procedure was used by which local AIDS service organisations were asked to recruit five to seven men who represent the diversity of the gay men they serve. The AIDS Service Organisations were chosen because they tend to have contact with men who would theoretically be most affected by ASS, given the hypothesis that level of contact to the disease is a predictor of having trauma symptoms. The resultant group of participants was diverse in terms of age (mean 32.4), education, professional status, and geographical region, reflecting patterns in larger epidemiological studies of gay men and HIV (for example, Bochow, 1994). Sixteen (24.6 per cent) of the men knew they were HIV-positive at the time of the interview; this is above the national prevalence for HIV among gay German men, which lies well below 10 per cent (Bochow, 1997).

There was a disproportionately large number of participants from cities with 500,000 or more residents. In spite of the sampling method, many of the men interviewed had only superficial contact to AIDS service structures.

Method

An exploratory study was undertaken in 1995–6 to test for the existence of an AIDS Survivor Syndrome among gay men in Germany. The leading hypothesis was that symptoms of trauma reactions could be found among men who have had the highest level of contact with the epidemic. The study was commissioned by the Department for Gay and Bisexual Men of the Deutsche AIDS-Hilfe, the National German AIDS Organisation.

Given the quality and scope of the instrument used in the New York study entitled 'Mental Health Effects of AIDS on At-Risk Homosexual Men', (Dean, undated) this questionnaire was requested from the researchers to be used as the basis for this investigation. The instrument was translated into German. To address potential problems due to cultural difference between the US and Germany and inappropriate formulations due to translation, the questionnaire was reviewed by three experts in the area of AIDS in Germany, two from the Deutsche AIDS-Hilfe and one noted researcher. Validity questions were further addressed through a pre-test of eight gay men from Berlin and from a smaller city. As a result of this process, the initial instrument was significantly shortened and some changes were made for the sake of clarity and cultural appropriateness. In making changes, careful attention was given to keeping sub-scales of the original intact so as not to threaten previously established reliability and validity.

The resultant interview lasted approximately two hours, taking place predominantly in participants' homes. All interviews were conducted personally by the investigator. Although largely quantitative in form, open-ended questions were also incorporated in the interview so as to address comprehensively twenty potential factors determining an AIDS Survivor Syndrome, essentially operationalising the hypothesized symptoms described above.

The various features of the syndrome were measured by employing several scales. Operationalising each of the hypothesized signs and symptoms listed above was not an easy task, given the lack of research in this area. A thorough description of this process has been published elsewhere. (See Wright, 1996.) In addition, qualitative information gathered during the course of the interviews was used to inform the interpretation of the data.

The hypothesis regarding the existence of ASS among the sample was tested by taking the existence of Post Traumatic Stress Disorder (PTSD) as being the dependent variable, using the rationale, based on existing literature, that at least these symptoms would need to be present to constitute a survivor syndrome. Appropriate tests of association were then calculated between PTSD and the other sub-scales of the instrument to test for the predicted relationships. Finally, a regression model was used to identify the constellation of factors best predictive of the PTSD symptoms.

Results

A comprehensive analysis of the data has been published elsewhere, essentially documenting the existence of the expected relationships (Wright, 1996). Interestingly, there was no evidence found that trauma symptoms predict putting oneself or others at risk for HIV infection. In the interest of space, we will focus here on the five factors in the analysis which were most highly correlated with the

PTSD scale. Given the small sample size, the number of variables entered into the regression equation needed to be limited. Using these five variables we will focus on the central question of whether or not the data gathered in this sample support the existence of an AIDS Survivor Syndrome among gay German men.

The five factors most correlated with PTSD symptoms were entered into a stepwise linear regression model, resulting in three factors explaining 75 per cent of the variance: having lost a partner or close friend to AIDS (0.43); denying the effects that AIDS has on one's life (0.40); and experiencing a general sense of demoralisation (0.29).[1] Being HIV-positive and having symptoms of sexual disturbance (impotency, lack of desire, etc.) are the other two factors most correlated with PTSD, but they do not contribute significantly to the regression model.

The absence of the HIV-positive variable in the regression equation does not, of course, mean that being positive is not significant in terms of developing trauma reactions. In addition to being associated with PTSD itself (0.35, $p < 0.005$), HIV is correlated with two variables in the regression model as well as with other markers of stress related to the epidemic, limiting the unique contribution of HIV status to the equation. (See Table 18.1.)

Discussion

The results of this exploratory study suggest that the AIDS Survivor Syndrome is a useful construct for describing the experience of gay men in response to the AIDS epidemic. Not only were symptoms of trauma found within the sample, but these symptoms were significantly associated with reactions which one would expect, given the existing literature on survivor syndromes; namely: demoralisation, having lost a partner or close friend to AIDS, denial of the effects that AIDS has on one's life, being HIV-positive and having symptoms of sexual disturbance.[2] In addition, three of these symptoms – denial, demoralisation and having lost a significant other to AIDS – predicted an impressive 75 per cent of the variance in the trauma reactions within the sample.

The results suggest that the lived experience of gay men in Germany places them at risk for developing symptoms of trauma, particularly those men whose contact with HIV/AIDS has been most immediate. According to survivor syndrome theory, the explanation for this finding is that being part of a community faced with a catastrophic threat, gay men can be overwhelmed by

Table 18.1 Correlations between being HIV-positive and other markers of AIDS-related stress

	Being HIV-positive
Having lost a partner or close friend to AIDS	0.49 (0.000)
Experiencing a general sense of demoralization	0.28 (0.043)
Total number of persons known living with HIV, weighted by level of intimacy	0.56 (0.000)
Total number of persons known who died from AIDS	0.36 (0.003)

issues such as grief, loss and their own illness. This produces symptoms which are not to be viewed as pathology, but rather as serious (and expected) reactions to extreme circumstances. (Compare Steinberg, 1989; Goderez, 1987; Fogelman, 1988.) Whether one actually develops trauma symptoms has been found to be related to the social support of the affected person; his/her pre-existing psychological strengths and weaknesses; his or her physical condition; as well as the circumstances under which he or she was exposed to the traumatic event (Davidson and Charny, 1993; Marcus and Rosenberg, 1988).

Many gay German men (particularly those living with HIV) are not only challenged by their own health concerns, but also by the sickness and death of those around them. Due to the social isolation of HIV-positive people and due to the confinement of the epidemic to specific segments of the population, the likelihood of someone who is gay (and particularly a gay man living with HIV) knowing men who are positive is higher, as compared to the general population. This, of course, results in these men being more likely to experience the death of people their own age who are fighting the disease.

Survivor syndrome theory offers a way of thinking about the experience of groups most effected by the AIDS epidemic which takes into account both the individual level of experience and the broader social environment in which that experience is lived. The traumatic effects of HIV are defined not only by the serious nature of the disease process itself, but also by the way it has ravaged relatively isolated and disadvantaged segments of the population, creating microclimates of suffering and death.

Of course, the findings of this research do not indicate that all gay German men are destined to develop trauma reactions due to the epidemic. The data do, however, suggest that men who have lived closest to the epidemic, and those who seek to help them, need to be particularly cognisant of the unusual stresses which they face. Given the role that denial seems to play in developing trauma symptoms, there is a particularly acute need to weigh realistically the events happening in one's life and to examine one's reactions to these events so as to develop an effective coping strategy.

This study was on a small scale and exploratory in nature. Due to limitations within the instrument, which was not originally designed to measure specifically ASS, and particularly due to small sample size, several relationships between variables could not be tested. This study does, however, provide sufficient evidence to pursue further research for which an instrument could be developed to measure more precisely ASS symptoms, allowing for studies of the prevalence and severity of ASS among populations of gay men, particularly within large epicentres, and providing data to describe in more detail the men most likely to be affected.

Conclusion

The findings of this exploratory study suggest that German gay men with immediate experience of the AIDS epidemic are at risk for developing symptoms of psychological trauma due to their experience with the disease. This distress is related not only to their own health status, but also to their social environment, which may be characterised by an unusual degree of sickness and death. The trauma reactions are also related to the degree these men seek to deny the effects AIDS is having on their lives.

These findings have implications particularly for the secondary prevention of HIV, that is for those programs designed to assist infected gay men and their significant others with the challenges of living with the disease. The survivor syndrome literature offers a way of understanding the experiences of these men, at both the individual level and within the societal context. This literature also offers several examples of successful interventions which can be adapted to address the needs of HIV-positive gay men (for example, Ochberg, 1991; Steinberg, 1989; Fogelman, 1988; Herbst, 1992; Catherall, 1986; for a summary of approaches see Wright, 1996). To meet the challenges of HIV disease, it is not only important that the specific circumstances of those affected by HIV be taken into account, but also that AIDS Service Organisations learn from the experience of other groups in society who have sought to cope with catastrophic events of a similar magnitude.

Notes

1   Beta coefficients (standardised regression coefficients) are given in parentheses for the variables in the equation.
2   Demoralisation is a measure of non-specific psychological symptoms which is sensitive to situations of extreme environmental distress, such as physical illness and catastrophic natural or man-made events. Communities undergoing such stressful experiences have been shown to have elevated demoralisation scores. A person is likely to develop demoralisation 'when he finds he cannot meet the demands placed on him by his environment, and cannot extricate himself from his predicament' (Frank, 1973: 316). (See Dean, undated; Dohrenwend *et al.*, 1979, 1980.)

References

Barrows, P. A. and Halgin, R. P. (1988) 'Current issues in psychotherapy with gay men: impact of the AIDS phenomenon', *Professional Psychology Research and Practice* (August) 19(4): 395–402.
Bochow, M. (1993) 'Einstellungen und Werthaltungen zu homosexuellen Männern in Ost- und Westdeutschland', in C. Lange (ed.), *Aids – eine Forschungsbilanz*, Berlin: edition sigma: 115–28.
—— (1994) *Schwuler Sex und die Bedrohung durch AIDS--Reationen homosexueller Männer in Ost- und Westdeutschland*, Berlin: Deutsche AIDS-Hilfe.
Bochow, M. (1997) *Schwule Männer und AIDS*, Berlin: Deutsche AIDS-Hilfe.
Catherall, D. R. (1986) 'The support system and amelioration of PTSD in Vietnam veterans', *Psychotherapy* 23(3): 472–82.
Dannecker, M. (1990) *Homosexuelle Männer und AIDS – eine sexualwissenschaftliche Studie zu Sexualverhalten und Lebensstil*, Stuttgart: Verlag W. Kohlhammer.
Davidson, A. G. (1991) 'Looking for love in the age of AIDS: the language of gay

personals, 1978–1988', *Journal of Sex Research* (February) 28(1): 125–37.

Davidson, S. and Charny, I. W. (1993) 'Recovery and integration in the life cycle of the individual and the collective', in S. Davidson, and I. W. Charny (eds), *Holding on to Humanity – The Message of Holocaust Survivors: The Shamai Davidson Papers*, San Francisco: Jossey-Bass: 189–210.

Dean, L. (undated) *Summary of Measures: Mental Health Effects of AIDS on At-Risk Homosexual Men*, New York: Columbia School of Public Health.

Deutsche AIDS-Hilfe (1993) Seminar 'Survivor Guilt', 2–3 October 1993, Berlin Konradshöhe, Berlin: Deutsche AIDS-Hilfe.

Dick, L. C. (1989) 'An investigation of the disenfranchised grief of two health care professionals caring for persons with AIDS', in K. J. Doka (ed.), *Disenfranchised Grief: Recognizing Hidden Sorrow*, Lexington, Mass.: Lexington/D. C. Heath: 55–65.

Dohrenwend, B. S. *et al.* (1979) *Report of the Public Health and Safety Task Force on Behavioral Effects to the President's Commission on the Accident at Three Mile Island* (Stock no. 052 – 003 – 00732 – 1), Washington, D.C.: US Government Printing Office.

Dohrenwend, B. S. *et al.* (1980) 'Nonspecific psychological distress and other dimensions of psychopathology: measures for use in the general population', *Archives of General Psychiatry* 37: 1229–36.

Doka, K. J. (1989) 'Disenfranchised grief', in K. J. Doka (ed.), *Disenfranchised Grief: Recognizing Hidden Sorrow*, Lexington, Mass.: Lexington/D. C. Heath: 3–11.

Eckstaedt, A. (1988) 'Eine klinische Studie zum Begriff der Traumareaktion. Ein Kindheitsschicksal aus der Kriegszeit', *Psyche* 34(7): 600–10.

Fogelman, E. (1988) 'Therapeutic alternatives for Holocaust survivors and second generation', in R. L. Braham (ed.), *The Psychological Perspectives of the Holocaust and of its Aftermath,* Boulder, Colo.: Social Science Monographs: 79–108.

Frank, J. D. (1973) *Persuasion and Healing*, Baltimore: Johns Hopkins Press.

Fuller, R. L., Geis, S. B. and Rush, J. (1989) 'Lovers and significant others', in K. J. Doka (ed.), *Disenfranchised Grief: Recognizing Hidden Sorrow*, Lexington, Mass.: Lexington/D. C. Heath: 33–42.

Giel, R. (1991) 'The psychosocial aftermath of two major disasters in the Soviet Union', *Journal of Traumatic Stress* 4(3): 381–92.

Goderez, B. I. (1987) 'The survivor syndrome: massive psychic trauma and posttraumatic stress disorder', *Bulletin of the Menninger Clinic* 51(1): 96–113.

Hakert, U. M. (1994) 'Wenn Überlebende sich schuldig fühlen', *Aktuell – Das Magazin der Deutschen Aids-Hilfe* (November) 8: 20–21.

Hays, R. B., Chauncey, S. and Tobey, L. A. (1990) 'The social support networks of gay men with AIDS', *Journal of Community Psychology* 18(4): 374–85.

Herbst, P. R. (1992) 'From helpless victim to empowered survivor: oral history as a treatment for survivors of torture', *Women and Therapy* 13(1–2): 141–54.

Jucovy, M. E. (1991) 'Psychoanalytic contributions to Holocaust studies', *International Journal of Psychoanalysis* 73: 267–82.

Klein, S. J. and Fletcher, W. (1986) 'Gay grief: an examination of its uniqueness brought to light by the AIDS crisis', *Journal of Psychosocial Oncology* 4(3): 15–25.

Krystal, H. and Niederland, W. G. (1968) 'Clinical observations on the Survivor Syndrome', in H. Krystal (ed.), *Massive Psychic Trauma*, New York: International Universities Press: 327–48.

Lennon, M. C., Martin, J. L. and Dean, L. (1990) 'The influence of social support on AIDS-related grief reaction among gay men', *Social Science and Medicine* 31(4): 477–84.

Marcus, P. R. and Rosenberg, A. (1988) 'A philosophical critique of the 'survivor syndrome' and some implications for treatment', in R. L. Braham (ed.), *The psychological Perspectives of the Holocaust and of its Aftermath*, Boulder, Colo.: Social Science Monographs: 53–73.

Martin, J. L. (1988) 'Psychological consequences of AIDS-related bereavement among gay men', *Journal of Consulting and Clinical Psychology* 56(6): 856–62.

Martin, J. L. and Dean, L. (1993) 'Effects of AIDS-related bereavement and HIV-related illness on psychological distress among gay men: a 7-year longitudinal study, 1985–1991', *Journal of Consulting and Clinical Psychology* 61(1): 94–103.

Martin, J. L., Dean, L., Garcia, M. and Hall, W. (1989) 'The impact of AIDS on a gay community: changes in sexual behavior, substance use, and mental health', *American Journal of Community Psychology* 17(3): 269–93.

Ochberg, F. M. (1991) 'Post-traumatic therapy', Special Issue: 'Psychotherapy with victims', *Psychotherapy* 28(1): 5–15.

Odets, W. (1995) 'In the shadow of the epidemic: being HIV-negative in the age of AIDS', Durham: Duke University Press.

Peters, U. H. (1989) 'Die psychischen Folgen der Verfolgung. Das Ueberlebenden-Syndrom. Fortschritte der Neurologie', *Psychiatrie* 57 (5): 169–91.

Pine, V. R. (1989) 'Death, loss, and disenfranchised grief', in K. J. Doka (ed.), *Disenfranchised Grief: Recognizing Hidden Sorrow*, Lexington, Mass.: Lexington /D. C. Heath: 13–23.

Schwartzberg, S. S. (1992) AIDS-related bereavement among gay men: the inadequacy of current theories of grief, *Psychotherapy* 29(3): 422–29.

Sklar, F. (1991) 'Grief as a family affair: property rights, grief rights, and the exclusion of close friends as survivors', *Omega Journal of Death and Dying*. 24(2): 109–21.

Steinberg, A. (1989) 'Holocaust survivors and their children: a review of the clinical literature', in P. Marcus and A. Rosenberg (eds) *Healing their Wounds: Psychotherapy with Holocaust Survivors and their Families*, New York: Praeger: 23–42.

Viney, L. L., Henry, R. M., Walker, B. M. and Crooks, L (1991) 'The psychosocial impact of multiple deaths from AIDS', *Omega Journal of Death and Dying* 24(2): 151–63.

Vogel, M. (1994) 'Wenn Schuld klinisch wird', *Aktuell – Das Magazin der Deutschen Aids-Hilfe* (November) 8: 22–3.

Wright, M. (1996) *Und wir überleben: Gibt es ein AIDS-Survivor-Syndrom unter schwulen Männern in Deutschland?* Berlin: Deutsche AIDS-Hilfe.

19 AIDS policy, health policy and gay politics

Rolf Rosenbrock

Introduction

Two theses and a rough description of their underpinnings will be presented in this chapter:

1 The implementation of AIDS policy in Germany pioneered success in terms of both health policy and gay politics. This approach to AIDS, implemented first in the former West Germany and then after 1990 in a unified Germany, mainly involved the fields of primary prevention, counselling and social support as well as the formation and networking of institutions.
2 In Germany today a gay movement hardly exists anymore in the sense of being a social movement. This is not due primarily to the successful AIDS policy itself, but rather to developments which the policy accelerated.

AIDS policy: starting point, implementation and content

The discovery in the mid-1980's of HIV and its paths of transmission revealed the social structure of the epidemic: not only the primarily affected groups but also the general public was threatened. In conjunction with the uncertain state of knowledge (which was much greater at the time) this triggered a great deal of fear throughout society. This fear had two forms: the fear of an unstoppable health catastrophe and the fear of new minority persecution. Both fears are understandable in retrospect. On the one hand, AIDS seemed to contradict an empirical principle that the age of infectious diseases was over in wealthy industrialised countries. On the other hand, in view of Germany's history of minority persecution, one had to reckon with strong tendencies in the direction of discrimination, exclusion and oppression. After all, the association of AIDS with sexuality, promiscuity, homosexuality, prostitution, drugs, addiction, crime, blood, death and HIV-infected persons as 'hidden enemies' brought together a sizeable bundle of volatile subjects.

The political debate thus had two issues rights from the start: health and civil rights. Confronted with such highly visible issues, not only the primarily affected groups but also all the forces in society normally concerned with health and civil rights homed in on the issue (Rosenbrock *et al.*, Chapter 20.) This combination of circumstances conferred a prominence to AIDS which, in comparison to other health risks, cannot be explained solely by the epidemiological danger. The interest was at times nothing short of hysterical. On the other hand, it also unleashed a great political willingness to tackle the problem.

Paradoxically, the political perception of the risk to society posed by AIDS was therefore productive, even though it was not necessarily rationally justified in terms of health policy. The extent and direction of the social reactions can only be understood as derivations of the health and civil rights policies from which they received their impetus.

A central actor in the political arena at this time was not in especially good shape compared to other European countries, namely the gay political movement in West Germany (Salmen and Eckert, 1989).[1] The great era of the movement's re-awakening at the time of the student revolts after 1968 drew to an end in the seventies. In about 1983 coalitions formed mainly in the larger cities consisting of activists from the 'old' gay movement as well as men who had usually not been actively involved in gay politics. The motive behind their actions was the threat posed to their lifestyle by AIDS. In a relatively short time these men founded a large number of regional AIDS Service Organisations (ASOs) based on foreign models, as well as the Deutsche AIDS-Hilfe (the National German AIDS Organisation) as their umbrella organisation. (See Schilling, Chapter 8.) The early organisers were viewed with distrust and even openly attacked by left-wing and apolitical gays who mainly saw in AIDS a dangerous tool of conservative moral policies, or simply an American problem (Bochow, 1993). The organisational weakness of the nascent ASO movement went unnoticed. The incipient political debate and the traditional role of associations in shaping policy in Germany required an actor such as an 'organisation of the primarily affected' as a partner. The extent to which the original organisers were themselves 'affected' by the disease was often faked in that small *adhoc* networks or *adhoc* groups were called on when the need arose (Paul, 1993).

The seductive power of the AIDS issue led to almost the entire gay political potential being mobilised for AIDS, with the exception of a few groups and active individuals who swam against the tide. So AIDS not only 'collectively trauma-tised' the gay community (Dannecker, 1990; Wright, Chapter 18), it also almost completely absorbed all visible gay political capacity. For the public at large, the topics of 'AIDS' and 'gayness' superimposed themselves in those years until they were nearly congruent.

The AIDS policy dispute from roughly 1984 to 1987, having both health policy and gay political elements, was multifaceted and sometimes bitter, focusing predominantly on the decisive medical and civil rights questions concerning the type of strategy to be employed against the impending pandemic (Rosenbrock, 1987; Rosenbrock and Salmen, 1990). Soon two, for the most part, mutually exclusive options arose. On the one side there was the classical epidemiological strategy based on the 'old public health' paradigm; that is, the individual search strategy that in American usage is called 'control and containment'. This approach is guided by the question: how do we quickly determine as many sources of infection as possible, and how do we shut them down? In contrast there was the 'new public health,' that is, a social learning strategy based on modern health science concepts, or 'inclusion and co-operation' in American usage. This approach searches for answers to the question: How can we quickly organise ongoing social learning processes on as broad a scale as possible in order to enable society to adjust to life with a presumably ineradicable virus without discriminating against those affected?

The debate was decided fairly quickly in favour of the learning strategy (Kirp and Bayer, 1992). In Germany, the political struggle was conducted more bitterly than in many other countries (Frankenberg and Hanebeck, Chapter 4) where there existed a richer and more untrammelled tradition of population-based health care (that is, public health), allowing them to display greater composure as compared to the Germans in their handling of sex, drugs and minorities. The outcome of this debate can, in retrospect, also be seen as a victory for rational health policy, having had good results in epidemiological terms and in respect to civil rights.

In the following I would like to discuss five aspects of the AIDS policy model that finally gained acceptance (compare Rosenbrock, 1994c) in order to outline the way AIDS policy, health policy and gay politics were related to each other (Rosenbrock, 1995). In this respect I understand gay politics to be efforts (if only modest) to reduce the social and legal discrimination of men who have sex with men. The following outline is intended to show that in AIDS policy there has been considerable overlap between health policy and policy aimed at the emancipation of male homosexuals. However, this overlap does not mean they are identical. To illustrate this point, I will compare the implications for health issues and gay politics within the AIDS policy model's central elements. Within this framework some of the deficits, inconsistencies and undesirable effects will receive less than their fair share of attention (Rosenbrock, 1992, 1994b, 1996).

Self-help and primary prevention

Health   Before AIDS the self-help movement was focused almost exclusively on the psychological, social, and medical aspects of coping with existing health problems, that is, on tertiary prevention (for example, alcoholism, cancer, seizure disorders, arthritis, obesity, bulimia). AIDS service groups, on the other hand, also worked for the prevention of the disease, that is, for primary prevention.

Homosexuality   This meant that homosexuality and homosexuals had acquired much greater social latitude and also a greater public acceptance. Gay lifestyles and relationships were talked about in public. This development has had both positive and negative consequences; but then nothing is without its undesirable effects.

Solidarity and public funding

Health   The vision often conjured up by public health researchers – namely, that of a spontaneous, solidarity-minded and self-organised coalition of people threatened by a common health risk – became a reality within the AIDS service movement (fortunately receiving significant amounts of public funding).

Homosexuality   This resulted in public resources being made available for gay projects, campaigns and institutions. It was possible to integrate a large number of gay working relationships and activities within the field of AIDS, and it was possible for gay men to champion their own cause. This had the price, of course, that homosexuality and AIDS became increasingly congruent in the public eye.

Success of community mobilisation

Health   The prevention campaigns were successful. Changes in attitudes and behaviour (see Bochow, Chapter 12; Dannecker, 1990) took place among the groups primarily affected by HIV risk, changes that exceeded prior results achieved in the history of public health (for example, personal hygiene, dental hygiene, smoking, drug use, etc.). Due to the mobilisation of cognitive, emotional and social resources in the target groups it was possible to influence areas of behaviour involving taboos, shame and illegal activity by way of publicly communicated learning. In principle, this is a success which could be expanded.

Homosexuality   In terms of gay politics this success is important not only because of homosexuals' surviving and living together as a group but also because it is a public shield against the preconceived notion that homosexuals are irresponsible and therefore must be handled with coercion and police measures. (See Jacob *et al.*, Chapter 9.)

Challenge to medical approaches of prevention

Health   The concepts and practice of the ASOs were based on a notion of health which did not relegate all responsibility for prevention and care to medicine. (See Etgeton, Chapter 7.) As a result, the first medical intervention for HIV, namely the HIV antibody test, was rejected as an inappropriate attempt to control an epidemic by focusing on the individual (Rosenbrock, 1994a).

Homosexuality   This challenge to medicine was of importance for gay politics because it ran counter to homophobic views of the compulsory identification of gay men as 'disease carriers'. With the rejection of the HIV antibody test as a tool of primary prevention, a new attempt to medicalise homosexuality was thwarted.

Health promotion and emancipation

Health   In keeping with more progressive health policy concepts, health means not only risk-avoiding behaviour but also the most autonomous life possible in self-chosen relationships and communities. The approach of the ASOs makes demands on both politicians and the larger social environment regarding improved living conditions in order to maximise health. The ASOs in their concrete structures provide their target groups with a place to realise this potential while fighting for change.

Homosexuality   The concept of health promotion, as set forth in the WHO Ottawa Charter, ties in to the emancipation of gay men, as well. The Charter states:

> Health promotion is the process of enabling people to increase control over, and to improve, their health. . . . Health is created and lived by people within the settings of their everyday life; where they learn, work, play and love. Health is created by caring for oneself and others, by being able to take decisions and have control over one's life circumstances, and by ensuring that the society one lives in creates conditions that allow the attainment of health by all its members.
>
> (WHO Ottawa Charter, 1986)

This somewhat literary sounding but, in terms of health policy, basically well-founded WHO declaration is officially supported by the German Federal Government. However, the statement is usually inconsequential since health promotion in this sense is addressed to everyone without naming any specific actors or concrete measures to be taken (Rosenbrock, 1997b). The Ottawa Charter only comes to life when it is cited by social and political movements to formulate their demands. In AIDS policy, this was done primarily by the ASOs which adopted central aspects of the Charter in the form of concepts like *structural prevention*. (See Etgeton, Chapter 7.) This built important bridges between health policy and gay politics, legitimising and promoting toleration and support for the gay subculture and related structures.

I would like to use six examples to elucidate the possibilities and limitations of the argument presented thus far:

1   Establishment of safer sex and the safer use norms presupposes a broad and multifaceted communication about these norms in the target groups. A reasonable health policy approach is, therefore, to promote this communication through preventing police intervention in the subcultures as well as through politically and financially supporting locations and structures of communication (for example, gay hotlines and information centres as found in Frankfurt/Main and Berlin).

2   If organisations formed by the primarily affected groups are identified as

central and irreplaceable actors in the AIDS prevention sector, any state
censure of their statements is incompatible with a targeted health policy.

3   If the marginal status of gay men and the resulting discrimination are
    viewed as an obstacle to co-operation and communication, then it is good
    health policy that a number of state governments in Germany have estab-
    lished official offices for homosexual issues.

4   If gay men in the process of coming out are identified as a group in
    particular need of AIDS prevention, then laws prohibiting homosexual sex
    are counterproductive in terms of health policy. Such laws result in men
    becoming illegally part of a community, so they are hard-to-reach and
    therefore more vulnerable. This argument played a significant role in the
    discussions leading to the repeal of Article 175 of the Penal Code in 1994
    which had been designed to punish homosexual acts.

5   Men who occasionally have sex with men, but who are not connected to
    gay communication structures, can be considered hard-to-reach in terms of
    AIDS prevention. The exclusion of gay encounters from educational
    messages designed for the general public (TV, movie theatres, print media,
    schools, etc.) cannot, therefore, be justified in terms of health policy. The
    Federal Centre for Health Education is doggedly working to implement the
    integration of such content in their national prevention campaigns. (See
    Pott, Chapter 6.)

6   If fidelity is propagated as a possible means of AIDS prevention, then the
    massive social, legal and financial discrimination of gay partnerships as
    compared to childless heterosexual married couples is illogical.

The AIDS policy approach described thus far made rapid progress possible in
terms of both health policy and gay emancipation, showing in exemplary fashion
what political difference is made by health policy rationale being combined with
a human rights movement. This is in contrast to the ongoing debate about
methadone maintenance for IV drug users and other forms of care challenging the
abstinence paradigm as well as HIV prevention in prisons. In other words there
has been much more support for the health policy demands made by the ASOs
regarding gay issues than for drug policies or the problems of prison inmates. It is
much easier to form an alliance of leftists, liberals, the gay lobby and gay organisations. This makes painfully clear the practical limits of alliances consisting of
the groups primarily affected by HIV and AIDS.

Virtually all political questions related to gay issues are represented by the
ASOs. This configuration is, however, beginning to crumble. For one, the ASOs
are gradually shifting their attention to the needs of gay men in socially under-
privileged life situations, reflecting larger epidemiological trends. (See Marcus,
Chapter 3; Bochow, Chapter 12.) The natural allies in serving this group are the
traditional Social Welfare Associations. (See Wright, Chapter 2.) For another, the
process of the ASOs having less gay personnel and less of a gay focus in general
is progressing rapidly, above all at the local level. There are now ASOs in which
gay men no longer hold any key positions.

Gay politics: consequences and outlook for the future

The achieving of gay political goals within the context of AIDS policy is viewed by some observers as being unquestionably positive. For example:

> With their AIDS service organisations the gay movement has taken an important step toward the institutionalisation of gay interests and has thus accelerated the integration of homosexuals in society.
>
> (Theis, 1997: 335)

Such a view is problematic for a number of reasons. It would be calamitous if the institutionalisation of gay interests coincided with HIV infection and the disease AIDS. There may be a broad overlapping of AIDS and gay issues, but that is far from their being identical. Today, being gay may surely include, personally and politically, an active participation in the prevention of HIV and solidarity with those infected. But that cannot be the full extent of gay politics.

Moreover, ASOs are not an unassailable bastion for gay issues. AIDS service organisations as an institution may well survive for a long time to come under more restrictive (and steadily deteriorating) socio-political conditions. But in the wake of the 'normalisation' of AIDS (Rosenbrock, 1994d; Rosenbrock et al., Chapter 20), the ASOs will increasingly lose their special status in respect to resources and attention. AIDS is a declining issue; the potential catastrophe has turned into a manageable public health problem. In the face of all reason and despite statements to the contrary (NAB, 1997), it is possible that sometime in the future medical treatment of the disease will degrade the standing of primary prevention in favour of a new dominance on the part of curative, individual-oriented medicine (Dannecker, 1997a). The introduction of home tests for HIV antibodies in Germany, temporarily averted in 1997, could undermine the counselling infrastructure of the ASOs (Rosenbrock, 1997a). For some time now the prevention work performed by the ASOs has also suffered from massive, unresolved problems of staffing which are of a structural and financial nature (Rosenbrock, 1996). The ASOs are also being constantly pushed and pulled in the direction of becoming less gay-oriented. They are also very dependent on money from the respective governmental body. This is to name just a few problems.

For these reasons, the ASOs cannot be a substitute for a gay political movement. Rather, they are a sort of health policy arm of organised homosexuals. The ASOs cannot achieve their goals without the personnel, material and lobby support of the gay community while at the same time they require a non-sectarian and pragmatic division of labour, because gay issues are not their only concern.

Against this background of the political experience gained through the German gay movement and AIDS policy it is necessary to pose three questions which will be briefly and provisionally touched on in the following:

1   Do we need a gay political movement?
2   Do we have a gay political movement?
3   If not, what do we have?

Do we need a gay political movement?

The need for a political movement can disappear if it loses its focus or if its issues have been worked through. In the case of gay politics there continue to be more than enough issues, for example:

- Distinct concepts of heterosexual normality still predominate in raising and educating children. As a result, the developmental issues facing children, youth and adults regarding their eventual coming out are often rendered unnecessarily difficult and sometimes life-threatening. Forms of sexuality other than heterosexuality must be communicated non-judgementally as accepted forms of living. This demand of the gay movement is surely increasingly capable of finding allies.
- Empirical studies point to a relatively stable baseline of gay discrimination and a willingness to discriminate against homosexuals (Dannecker, 1997b). Today, an established intellectual in a large city would not be subject to such treatment, but the class-specific and urban/rural differences are considerable.
- Equal legal standing is still not existent for gay and heterosexual couples with respect to insurance, taxes, inheritance, pension, visiting rights in the case of sickness, the refusal to testify against one's partner, housing, and general business practices.
- The commercialisation of nearly all forms of gay life is leading to cultural and habitual patterns and to a selectivity that are enriching while at the same time inhibiting the possibilities of an unimpeded, general communication between gay men.[2] Since every social movement also develops its own milieu, a considerable enrichment of gay culture would be expected from a political gay movement.[3]
- Despite the apparently long-term success achieved regarding AIDS, it is never possible to rule out the danger of a backlash, for example, a 'new Puritanism' in the form of a populist social envy of 'people who refuse to raise children' or of 'double income, no kids' couples, or in reaction to another unforeseeable event analogous to AIDS.
- Finally, in international comparison, gays in Germany live on one of the few isles of the blest, in regard to the legal, material and political conditions in the country. In nearly half of all countries in the world gays and lesbians are denied basic human rights (Herzer, 1997). Political activity at an international level can, therefore, still find many issues to address.

So there are still enough gay political issues at hand, particularly the kinds of issues requiring the intervention of a social movement. There are also no signs that these issues are disappearing any time soon. Even the most elaborate discussions between essentialists and constructivists as well as all the reports and speculation about new predilections or even 'new sexualities' in ever more distinct subcultures cannot detract from the fact that a certain number of men and women feel attracted to their own gender in a more or less stable erotic, sexual or emotional way and that the acceptance or fulfilment of this desire encounters a number of social obstacles.

Do we have a gay political movement?

A lot of actors in the political realm naturally claim to be the legitimate representatives of the gay movement. Such claims must, of course, be assessed less by the success of their public relations than by concepts of what constitutes a social movement. In keeping with Dieter Rucht (1994: 77):

> [A] social movement . . . [is] . . . an active system based on a mobilised network of groups and organisations set up for a certain period of time and supported by a collective identity. This network seeks to bring about, prevent, or rescind social change by means of protest, including the use of force where necessary. Social change in this context means a fundamental change in the social order. . . . Essentially, if not explicitly, the movement focuses on basic structures of economic regulation, political power, and the setting of socio-cultural norms. The utopian ideas of social movements in particular provide information on the potential range of the intended changes.

No matter how keenly one may search in Germany, any collective example of gay politics would at most meet only a few of the criteria contained in this definition. The utopian idea of a solidarity-minded and also sexually liberated society, the precondition for which would be an overcoming of capitalism and patriarchy, does not for now appear to be have a broad effect, or to be capable of finding allies.

Another criterion is not addressed in Rucht's definition; that is, social movements customarily organise their own social milieu. That was true of the gay movement in the 1970s. It still holds true to only a very limited extent for existing homosexual organisations like the Association of Lesbians and Gays in Germany (LSVD). Like many other areas of society, this sole national association is moving in the direction of becoming a service provider and lobby with a pragmatic focus on reducing social and legal inequality, usually in the form of planned single-purpose campaigns. Current examples include the public relations work on 'gay marriage' and the issue of violence against gays. Such work is necessary and meritorious, but it is not a campaign of a social movement. The reason for this difference or deficit is the fact that the organisations in charge simply are not at the same time the organisers of the social milieu. There will not be any great change as long as homosexual men satisfy their needs for 'milieu' in the various commercialised scenes. A consequence, however, is the decline in the ability to mobilise and thus to conduct campaigns. This is, so to speak, the price of integration.

So what does that leave us with?

The assessment thus far may seem excessively pessimistic. At the same time, the expanded gay presence as a reward for integration cannot be overlooked. Next to lobbies like the LSVD there is an open presence of gays in political organisations, parliaments, trade unions, the media and science. Many new and autonomous but poorly networked gay centres are developing. Tentative attempts are also being made to organise bisexuals; and naturally there are the fairly unspectacular but tenacious traditional associations like the network Homosexuals and the Church (HuK). Utopian ideas to provide orientation and mobilisation while being capable of attracting allies – ideas pointing beyond civil rights and thus giving rise to completely new issues and alliances – are nowhere to be seen.

It is in any case obvious that two segments of organised gay life are expanding the most. For one, the gay market segment, both as the addressee of ostensibly provocative advertising messages and in the form of a growing number of gay businesses. The latter includes gay yellow pages in which the gay man can shop so that the 'money stays in the family' (sic!). For another, gay leisure activities, above all sports and singing, probably have more members than all gay political groups put together (Hinzpeter, 1997). Despite a sometimes annoyingly uncritical attitude toward commercial sponsorship, etc., this is for the most part a welcome development, an indication of the public mobility of gays.

In respect to open gay political problems and latent threats, there is, of course, the question whether gay business, leisure activities, lobbies, and gay segments in other areas of society can adequately mobilise for the political and social emancipation of gay men. One can have doubts. As examples, I have chosen two issues related to AIDS for which, in my view, gay involvement was called for but was hardly seen.

When in the autumn of 1993, that is, long after the end of AIDS hysteria, a kind of blanket testing of the population for HIV was briefly considered in the course of the blood contamination scandal (compare Rosenbrock, 1995; Frankenberg and Hanebeck, Chapter 4), there was nothing to be seen or heard from gay organisations apart from a few press statements.

When in the spring of 1997 the funds for the Deutsche AIDS-Hilfe were dropped for its public relations and international affairs departments, both essential for AIDS work and gay politics, there was only feeble protest to be heard from the ASOs themselves and from a few solidarity-minded journalists. There was virtually nothing to be heard or felt in the way of political protest, the formation of alliances, or even gay resistance. The minimal obligation of the gay community to the ASOs, their 'health policy arm' was not honoured. It is hard to judge whether these two examples were merely exceptions, though highly significant in themselves, or whether they mark a long-term trend.

Conclusion

In summary, there is currently nothing to be seen of a gay movement in Germany in the sense of a social movement. ASOs and other organisations that have formed around this plague have occasionally assumed that role and have concentrated political resources for themselves. This was necessary, successful, and therefore also appropriate. But in the long run, this construction will not stand the test. Too many gay issues will be ignored politically.

Notes

1   Female homosexuality, which has been affected in very different ways by AIDS, is not discussed in this chapter.
2   Regarding the different forms of communication and styles of association in the former East Germany see Rosenbrock and Herrn, 1996 as well as Herrn, Chapter 13.
3   The fact cannot be overlooked that AIDS Service Organizations have produced notable innovations within the scope of the structural prevention concept. The ASOs have succeeded not only in protecting but also shaping 'gay habitats'.

References

Bochow, M. (1993) 'Reactions of the gay community to AIDS in East and West Berlin', in *Aspects of AIDS and AIDS-Hilfe in Germany*, AIDS-Forum DAH, vol. 12, Berlin: Deutsche AIDS Hilfe: 19–45.

Bochow, M. (1997) *Schwule Männer und AIDS. Eine Befragung im Auftrag der Bundeszentrale für gesundheitliche Aufklärung 1996, AIDS-Forum DAH*, Berlin: Deutsche AIDS-Hilfe.

Dannecker, M. (1990) *Homosexuelle Männer und AIDS. Eine sexualwissenschaftliche Studie zu Sexualverhalten und Lebensstil, Schriftenreihe des Bundesministeriums für Jugend, Familie, Frauen und Gesundheit Band 252*, Stuttgart, Berlin and Cologne: Verlag W. Kohlhammer.

Dannecker, M. (1997a) *Das andere AIDS. AIDS Infothek*, vol. 9, Issue 3: 4–7.

—— (1997b) *Deutschland – ein schwulenfreundliches Land? Zeitschrift für Sexualforschung*, 10: 229–32.

Hegener, W. (1997) 'Von der schwulen Identität, die nicht aufhört aufzuhören', in E. Kraushaar (ed.) *Hundert Jahre schwul. Eine Revue*, Berlin: Rowohlt Verlag: 219–33.

Herzer, M. (1997) 'Verfolgung und Widerstand weltweit', in Schwules Museum/Akademie der Künste (ed.), *Goodbye to Berlin. 100 Jahre Schwulenbewegung*, Berlin: Verlag rosa Winkel: 340–41.

Hinzpeter, W. (1997) *Schöne schwule Welt. Der Schlußverkauf einer Bewegung*, Berlin: Querverlag.

Jacob, R., Eirmbter, W. H. et al. (1997) *AIDS-Vorstellungen in der Bevölkerung. Ergebnisse sozialwissenschaftlicher AIDS-Forschung Band 18*, Berlin: edition sigma.

Kirp, D. and Bayer, R. (eds) (1992) *AIDS in Industrial Democracies:Passions, Politics, and Policies*, New Brunswick, N.J.: Rutgers University Press.

Kraushaar, E. (ed.) (1997) *Hundert Jahre schwul. Eine Revue*, Berlin: Rowohlt Verlag.

NAB (Nationaler AIDS-Beirat) (1997) *Votum 35: AIDS-Prävention vor dem Hintergrund knapper Haushaltsmittel, 5 May 1997*, unpublished manuscript, Bonn: BMG.

Paul, G. (1993) 'Vorstände von 1983 bis 1993 über ihre Arbeit und die Entwicklung der D.A.H.', in Deutsche AIDS-Hilfe (ed.), *10 Jahre Deutsche AIDS-Hilfe. Geschichte und Geschichten, AIDS-Forum D.A.H. Special edition*, Berlin: Deutsche AIDS-Hilfe: 60–7.

Rosenbrock R. (1987) 'Some social and health policy requirements for the prevention of AIDS', *Health Promotion* 2(2): 161–8.

—— (1992) *AIDS: Fragen und Lehren für Public Health. Jahrbuch für kritische Medizin 18: Wer oder was ist Public Health?* Hamburg: Argument-Verlag: 82–114.

—— (1994a) 'Der HIV-Test ist die Antwort – aber auf welche Fragen?' in R. Rosenbrock, H. Kühn and B. M. Köhler (eds), *Präventionspolitik. Gesellschaftliche Strategien der Gesundheitssicherung*, Berlin: edition sigma: 358–82.

—— (1994b) 'Public Health: AIDS als Paradigma?' in W. Zapf and M. Dierkes (eds), *Institutionenvergleich und Institutionendynamik, WZB-Jahrbuch*, Berlin: edition sigma: 159–81.

—— (1994c) 'Strategie und Politik für wirksame AIDSprävention', *AIDS-Forschung (AIFO)* 9(2): 85–90.

—— (1994d) *Die Normalisierung von AIDS – teils nach vorne, teils zurück*, ed. D. Kirp and R. Bayer: 480–501.

—— (1995) 'AIDS – Gesundheit und Homosexualität. Allgemeine und aktuelle Bemerkungen zum Verhältnis zweier Diskurse', in *Homosexualität, AIDS und Menschenrechte. In Memoriam Siegfried R. Dunde*, Cologne: Deutsche AIDS Stiftung o.J.: 259–76.

—— (1996) 'Sind neue Erkenntnisse zu Risikokonstellationen präventionspolitisch umsetzbar?', in H. Jäger (ed.), *AIDS – Management der Erkrankung, Landsberg*: ecomed: 389–92.

—— (1997a) 'Welche Verbesserungen kann der HIV-Home Sampling Test bringen?', *Infektionsepidemiologische Forschung* 2: 40–3.

—— (1997b) 'Hemmende und fördernde Faktoren in der Gesundheitspolitik – Erfahrungen aus dem vergangenen Jahrzehnt', in T. Altgeld, I. Laser, and U. Walter (eds), *Wie kann Gesundheit verwirklicht werden? Gesundheitsfördernde Handlungskonzepte und gesellschaftliche Hemmnisse*, Weinheim and Munich: Juventa Verlag.

Rosenbrock, R. and Herrn, R. (1996) *Kommunikationsstrukturen, Gesellungsstile und Lebensweisen schwuler Männer in den neuen Bundesländern, Forschungsantrag*, unpublished manuscript, Berlin: WZB.

Rosenbrock, R. and Salmen, A. (eds) (1990) *AIDS Prävention. Ergebnisse sozialwissenschaftlicher AIDS-Forschung Band 1*, Berlin: edition sigma.

Rucht, D. (1994) *Modernisierung und neue soziale Bewegungen*, Frankfurt/Main and New York: Campus Verlag.

Salmen, A. and Eckert, A. (1989) *20 Jahre bundesdeutsche Schwulenbewegung, 1969 – 1989, BVH-Materialien 1*, Cologne: Bundesverband Homosexualität.

Schwules Museum/Akademie der Künste (ed.) (1997) *Goodbye to Berlin. 100 Jahre Schwulenbewegung*, Berlin: Verlag rosa Winkel.

Theis, W. (1997) 'AIDS – oder die teuer erkaufte Professionalisierung der Schwulenbewegung', in Schwules Museum/Akademie der Künste (ed.), *Goodbye to Berlin. 100 Jahre Schwulenbewegung*, Berlin: Verlag rosa Winkel: 327–35.

WHO (1986) *Ottawa Charter for Health Promotion*, Geneva: World Health Organisation.

Part V

The future of AIDS policy and practice

20 The normalisation of AIDS in Germany

Rolf Rosenbrock, Doris Schaeffer and Martin Moers

Introduction: AIDS on the path from exceptionalism to normality

As several articles in this volume attest, the crisis caused by the AIDS epidemic in Germany has abated. An impending catastrophe has turned into a problem that can be managed by public health and medical care. For this reason there is talk of the 'end of exceptionalism' (Bayer, 1991) and of 'normalisation' (Schaeffer *et al.*, 1992). Integration into evolved routines, regulations and institutions, that is into the 'normally poor course of health policy' (Rosenbrock, 1986) is, of course, not a seamless process or one free of contradictions. That is due, above all, to the fact that the outbreak of AIDS attracted not only special attention in Germany but also led to a high degree of readiness to try out innovative processes as well as to disburse large amounts of money. AIDS became the exception to many rules in health policy, prevention and patient care. People saw in these innovations not only an appropriate response to the challenge posed by HIV to health and health policy but also the opportunity for the long overdue testing of new forms of social management for other health risks (Rosenbrock, 1993).

Generally, normalisation entails risks and opportunities (Rosenbrock, 1994a) and is a contradictory process. In the case of AIDS, this process involves not only measures related directly to HIV but also to modernisation trends in the field of health policy (prevention and patient care) and with respect to society as a whole. To understand this process and to assess these risks and opportunities it is helpful to distinguish between four phases in the social and political response to AIDS (van den Boom, 1998):

Phase I (c. 1981–6): the emergence of exceptionalism During this period, HIV/AIDS made its debut. Public policy needed to be conceptualised, decided on and implemented. In some cases, the initial policies were institutionalised, but with a high degree of uncertainty. This was a time of considerable political tension and of short time frames for action. AIDS triggered a high degree of political readiness for innovation and resource allocation.

Phase II (c. 1986–91): the consolidation of exceptionalism The ways of working, the newly defined roles, and the institutional structures that arose in the context of exceptionalism began to consolidate. At the same time, it became increasingly clear that gay men and IV drug users would remain the most affected groups in the near term, as well. Catastrophic changes in terms of incidence and prevalence did not take place. Nevertheless, AIDS retained its unchallenged special status.

Phase III (c. 1991–6): exceptionalism diminishing, steps toward normalisation
Persistently stable epidemiological trends were accompanied by a calmer debate concerning minorities and civil rights. Therapeutic success resulted in AIDS taking on a chronic pattern, leading to the first erosion of the disease's special status and to cut backs in the resources invested in combating the epidemic. At the same time, the management of AIDS was consolidated and professionalised.

Phase IV (since 1996): normalisation   Due in part to successful prevention, new HIV infections and AIDS cases have reached an epidemiological equilibrium far below the levels feared. (See Marcus, Chapter 3.) The alliance between health care professionals and social movements dealing with AIDS is revealing signs of fatigue. New anti-retroviral therapies have extended survival dramatically, while at the same time market-oriented cost containment policies have gained acceptance. Some of the innovations in prevention and care achieved with exceptionalism are being called into question, while others have been integrated into the normal course of policy making, administration, prevention, and health care.

Phase I (*c.* 1981–6)

The reasons for exceptionalism

To understand the extent of the innovations linked to exceptionalism it is necessary to remember what led to a broad consensus in Germany that HIV/AIDS could not simply be countered with the routine repertoire of health policy. This consensus was reached by affirming the responsibility of the State for public health intervention as well as the long-standing policy of a non-discriminatory access to state-of-the-art health care.

A survey of national studies on the policy trend toward exceptionalism (Kirp and Bayer, 1992; Setbon, 1993; Lichtenstein, 1997; Ballard, 1998; Cattacin, 1996, 1998; van den Boom, 1998) paints a picture of several inter-related aspects of health policy, civil rights and social policy which explain both the extent and direction of the innovations undertaken. These aspects, detailed below, apply to the German situation, as well.

With the extensive availability of effective antibiotics since the 1940s there was, in general, widespread certainty that the age of infectious diseases had come to an end in wealthy, industrialised countries. The emergence of HIV and AIDS thus had a lasting, unsettling impact on this conviction. It also soon became clear that clinical medicine was powerless over HIV and that it would remain so for a long time to come. The deep belief in the ability of medicine to guarantee health suffered a severe setback, not only for the public at large, but also for members of the health care professions themselves.

HIV is mainly transmitted by unprotected sexual intercourse, especially anal intercourse, and by sharing contaminated needles during drug use. These means of transmission, as well as the continued infectivity during the long period of latency, touched on many social taboos and thus activated archaic fears among the public. As a consequence, the political climate was very charged (Frankenberg, 1992; Frankenberg and Hanebeck, Chapter 4). In addition, the decisions about health policy had to be made in a phase in which there was hardly any certainty about the extent of the threat, that is, the efficiency of transmission, the reliability and acceptance of protective strategies, etc. As not only IV drug users but also the entire, sexually-active population appeared to be at serious risk, the willingness to take unaccustomed measures was increased.

The ineffectiveness of 'old public health' as applied to STDs was also an important topic. Compulsory examinations, screenings, strict rules of behaviour, restricting civil rights (including large scale invasions of privacy), as well as quarantines, contact tracing and compulsory therapy had proven to be epidemiologically effective only under very special and politically irreproducible conditions (for example, in armies with state-controlled prostitution; Brandt, 1987). The greater the doubt was about the effectiveness and efficiency of conventional measures for the prevention of contagious diseases (especially STDs), the more the readiness to try new approaches grew. The decision against 'old public health' was in the case of AIDS easier to make because, in contrast to past epidemics, elements of an alternative strategy were already available, at both the conceptual level and in the form of numerous practical approaches; for example, public campaigns to reduce cardiovascular risks and various methods of influencing behaviour change which had been developed since the 1960s (Puska *et al.*, 1985; Farquhar *et al.*, 1990; Ballard, 1998). This arsenal of approaches paved the way for new risk management strategies in responding to AIDS. The basic model of preventing disease through education and information achieved the status of a worldwide consensus in the form of the WHO Ottawa Charter for Health Promotion (WHO, 1986).

The choice of a strategy based on an educational model was also attractive politically because it made possible the inclusion and instrumentalisation of social movements that had arisen in response to AIDS. Most importantly, the gay community had begun to organise behavioural change in their own ranks and had been calling for the support of the larger society and for legal protection of the freedoms the gay liberation movement had achieved since the 1960s. (See Schilling, Chapter 8; Rosenbrock, Chapter 19.) Thus, there was social impetus, in the form of political pressure, for a type of intervention based on mobilisation and activism, and there was support in society in the form of a great readiness to become engaged and take action (for example, through volunteering).

In summary: the occurrence of AIDS in Germany opened up a 'window of opportunity' (Kingdon, 1984) for new approaches and projects in health policy of a magnitude that is extraordinarily rare. In the phases to follow, several new elements of policy were realised in Germany as a result.

Phase II (c. 1986–91)

From exceptionalism to a model case in modern health policy

The synthesised 'complete' model of the way in which AIDS was handled in Germany has become known as exceptionalism and can be summarised in five interdependent complexes:[1]

Policy formulation procedure   As described by Frankenberg and Hanebeck (Chapter 4) the fundamental political questions raised by AIDS were debated publicly – sometimes in a very controversial fashion – and negotiated in an open political system between NGOs, governments, and various professional groups. This democratic/participatory process created in an unusually short period of time a very high level of information and an elevated public consciousness. In this respect, the process can be viewed as being a relatively successful example of public risk communication, and thus of the discursive definition and assessment of a social risk (Cattacin, 1998).

Actor configuration in policy formulation and implementation   In both the formulation and implementation of policy there were considerable deviations in regard to both the circle of actors involved and the distribution of power and responsibility between the actors as compared to the management of other health risks. (See Frankenberg and Hanebeck, Chapter 4.) The otherwise strong role played by medicine was weakened because effective treatment of the HIV infection was not available and mass screenings using the HIV antibody test were viewed as incompatible with the prevention model. In the field of patient care, hitherto under-rated health professionals (nurses, psychologists, social workers) as well as actors in the field of outpatient care gained influence and importance *vis-à-vis* the hospital sector. Organisations of the groups mainly affected by the disease, above all gay men, assumed roles in the field of patient care to a previously unknown extent

Policy formulation and implementation in primary prevention   Building on experience gained with community-related prevention and health promotion as well as on the WHO Ottawa Charter, a new prevention concept was developed. The concept called for influencing the social environment to strengthen people's motives for preventive behaviour and to weaken motives for taking risk. This was in opposition to approaches which sought to change people's conduct through coercion or by simply distributing information. The concept became known in Germany as *structural prevention*. (See Etgeton, Chapter 7.) Based on this idea, only appropriate channels of communications were used on three aggregate levels (national population-based campaigns, community-specific campaigns, personal counselling). The three levels were co-ordinated in the interest of furthering non-contradictory educational messages. (See Pott, Chapter 6.) This approach to the prevention of a mainly sexually transmitted disease represents a transition from a 'despotic' and individualised direct control to 'infrastructural', population-based indirect control (Mann, 1986). In other words, it is a move from the 'control and containment' approach to that of 'inclusion and co-operation' (Bayer, 1989) and from an 'individual search strategy' to a 'public learning strategy' (Rosenbrock, 1987).

Policy formulation and implementation in health care   The professional health-care system initially displayed defensive reactions, including denying AIDS patients treatment. Structural changes in patient care were finally rendered possible through the initially strong support of health care professionals (physicians, nurses, psychologists and social workers). These changes were already underway for the treatment of chronic diseases more generally, but the process lacked wider recognition. These advances in the field of care were aimed primarily at improving quality of life and making a patient-orientated approach the central guiding principle. Special community-based nursing services as well as medical practices specialising in HIV and AIDS and others specialising in the controlled administration of methadone were established (Moers and Schaeffer, 1992a; see also Schaeffer, Chapter 17).

Screening policy and risk assessment   The HIV antibody test in 1984 provided a technical tool for determining a person's serostatus. The purpose of the test and the extent and context for its use comprised a central contested topic in the negotiation of AIDS policy in Germany. The effects of exceptionalism on AIDS screening is seen in the definition of the test's objectives. There were well-substantiated reasons for not instituting mass screenings and a compulsory use of the test for primary prevention (Rosenbrock, 1991, 1994b). This led to both political and scientific disputes which called secondary preventive approaches into question (early detection for the purpose of medical and behavioural intervention) – not only in regard to AIDS, but in regard to other diseases, as well (Holland and Stewart, 1990; Abholz, 1994; Miller and Lipman, 1996). The result of this debate was the recommendation that the test be widely recommended to those at risk only in the case that medical treatment become available which had a heightened efficacy if initiated during the symptom-free phase of the disease. (Compare Rosenbrock, 1986.)

To summarise: if, as done here, the primary elements are put together to form an 'ideal' overall picture for the national AIDS policy in Germany, it can be seen that it was possible to realise numerous innovations at every stage of the public health action cycle – innovations that in earlier years could not be pushed through because of 'reform blockades in the health system' (Rosewitz and Webber, 1990). The further fate of this model and its role in the process of normalisation is therefore of significance to health policy and to the health sciences far beyond the AIDS phenomenon.

Phase III (*c.* 1991–6)

The forces driving normalisation

Normalisation designates a process in which a phenomenon that was previously considered as extraordinary loses this status and returns to the world of the familiar and customary in terms of both perception and action. As a result, public attention declines or is restricted to a specific issue community. At the end of the process, deviation from the general rule (in the form of exceptionalism), is neutralised. The forces driving the normalisation of AIDS are of different types and can be categorised as having non-specific and AIDS-specific causes.

Non-specific causes of normalisation

Basically, societies display a remarkable potential to come to terms with new risks and, in this sense, to normalise them. People grow accustomed to various natural, technical, economic, social and political phenomena as society begins to treat the associated issues 'normally' through processes of mutual agreement and definition (Cattacin, 1998). The 'issue attention cycle' (Downs, 1972) describes the course taken by this sometimes frighteningly capacious ability of individuals, groups and societies to adjust to serious situations simply by neglecting them.

At the same time, other topics start to elbow their way to the fore and over-shadow the explosiveness of the problem once viewed as extraordinary. The fear of AIDS as an infectious disease was, for instance, overshadowed or relativised by the repeated emergence of Ebola epidemics, the flare-up of cholera in India, BSE in Europe, the chicken virus in Hong Kong, etc. This is not to mention the more common infectious diseases having regained attention due to AIDS – such as tuberculosis and malaria – that are continuing almost unchecked in poor countries.

At the level of direct service staff in prevention and patient care, the waning of public attention has had the consequence of diminished motivation to continue working. This is due in part to the difficulty in maintaining the extremely high levels of commitment found in times of exceptionalism, given the workers' reliance on social gratification (Ullrich, 1987; Aust, 1996). When public attention declines, the gratification potential disappears and thus one of the central well-springs for regeneration of personal motivation dries up (Schaeffer *et al.*, 1992).

Exceptionalism always requires extraordinary solutions and innovative action. The transition to normalisation requires the ability to integrate these changes. The first steps toward integration are tantamount to a cross-roads. Many founding members of organisations leave the field or make their way into other fields or positions. The transition from exceptionalism to normalisation is, as a consequence, usually linked to changes in the configuration of actors. Many new staff members bring with them other coping attitudes as well as other motivations which are often distinguished less by altruism than by professional interest. The new staff are thus inspired less by utopian ideals than by realistic imperatives (Schaeffer *et al.*, 1992).

In Western industrialised societies the management of risks, including AIDS, is often given a nudge by social movements. The society's response to risk thus reflects all the characteristic twists and turns of these movements (Rucht, 1994). This includes the pattern of topics exhausting themselves once the actors in the exceptionalist alliance turn to emerging issues, or to issues which have not lost their public appeal. Consistent with this tendency is the way in which AIDS strengthened the self-help movement in Germany and how this movement is now undergoing the process of transformation from informal structures to formal institutions. This has altered the nature of the NGOs to the extent that they 'normalise' themselves by becoming an integral part of the welfare state and are subject to its functions (Rosenbrock, 1994a). This process of transformation of NGOs is generally tied to a de-politicising of the issue.

AIDS-specific causes of normalisation

While exceptionalism was based largely on the fact that medicine was on the defensive, the first biomedical successes have since been documented. Due to improved knowledge and a larger number of therapeutic possibilities, AIDS is increasingly becoming a manageable disease. Medicine once again is becoming a decisive player in the struggle against HIV. A reconfiguration of the actors has ensued, with other health professions (for example, nursing and social work) again losing their importance and their ability to shape events.

With the growth in therapeutic possibilities AIDS is increasingly perceived and managed as a chronic condition, displaying all the structural features of this type of illness (longevity, long course of events, inconstancy) and thus taking its place in the spectrum of today's dominant group of diseases in wealthy countries (Fee and Fox, 1992). We see how the course of the disease has changed when comparing the average survival time for an AIDS diagnosis in Germany in 1998 (8.9 months) with the average survival time in 1996 (just prior to the availability of combination therapies: 20.1 months; Hamouda *et al.*, 1997; see also Marcus, Chapter 3).

Whereas during the phase of exceptionalism AIDS triggered a great willingness to take action and invest resources; we notice a decline in the readiness of actors in the government and health care system to enter into political and financial commitments regarding AIDS. For example, the Federal Centre for Health Education has been subjected to significant cut backs over time. (See Pott, Chapter 6.)

Many pioneers committed themselves to AIDS because the disease posed a concrete threat to them and those in their environment. The constant confrontation with death and dying has led to overload and burn-out phenomena (Moers and Schaeffer, 1992b; Kleiber *et al.*, 1995; Bayer and Oppenheimer, 1998). Especially in the NGOs, but also in many of the care facilities specialising in AIDS, it is not only the death of clients and patients which characterised the everyday work, but also the loss of many committed activists to the disease.

Phase IV (since 1996)

Normalisation: preliminary results and perspectives

In comparison to the AIDS health policy model that made exceptionalism possible, the current reality presents a contradictory picture as a result of normalisation processes drawing to a close. AIDS-related task forces and specific government agencies are being cut back or (re-)integrated into the normal hierarchic/bureaucratic structures (Cattacin, 1998). Some of the resources for prevention and research are also being drastically reduced. Such cutbacks are a justifiable response to declining demand and to the overestimated magnitude of the epidemic. This scaling down is, however, often being done at the expense of prevention efficacy and quality of care (that is, normalisation in the form of cut backs). At the same time, many AIDS-related innovations have gained acceptance and have become institutionalised (that is, normalisation in the service of stabilising the exceptionalism). Finally, AIDS has also launched developments which have been so successful as to become new norms for general practice (that is, normalisation as a generalisation of exceptionalism).

Examples of stabilisation, cutbacks, and generalisation as well as numerous mixed forms are to be found in all of the policy fields touched by AIDS. Below are examples from three policy fields strongly shaped by the disease: patient care, primary prevention and drug use.

AIDS patient care: normalisation in the midst of innovation and medicalisation

In the care of people with HIV and AIDS exceptionalism brought forth a large number of successful reforms with implications for patient care more generally. Several directions are emerging as we observe these innovations being revoked in certain cases, consolidated in others, and applied to other areas of care. There are several noteworthy aspects of this process, for example:

- As therapeutic possibilities grow, the focus on patient-orientated care has lessened. In other words, there has been a shift in priorities from care to cure.
- In the course of this development medicine has reclaimed the power to define and shape HIV policies and has recouped the external resources it appeared to have lost for a number of years.[2] As a consequence, other health professions (nurses, psychologists, social workers, etc.) and community organised services are, once again, losing importance.
- Many innovations in health care owe their existence to the commitment of well-organised, middle-class AIDS patient interest groups who asserted their right to appropriate care. In the case of other groups – for example, members of the lower classes, immigrants and, above all, IV drug users – one can see deficits in care due to a lack of advocacy (Schaeffer, 1995a, 1995b; Luger, 1998).

- Despite the severity of HIV disease, care is provided primarily on an outpatient basis. The outpatient sector found it difficult to fill adequately the position that had devolved upon it (Moers and Schaefer, 1998; Schaeffer, 1996) due in part to the underdevelopment of professional nursing and infrastructural deficits in the field of home care in Germany. (See Schaeffer, Chapter 17.)
- For people with HIV and AIDS normalisation mainly means a longer life, but with the price of the disease becoming a chronic problem. As a result, a shift can be seen in the priorities of those affected. Where during the period of exceptionalism maximum priority was attached to surviving, mundane problems of living with HIV and AIDS now have a far higher standing.

AIDS prevention: between fatigue, retreat and expansion to other areas of health care

The primary prevention of HIV is probably one of the most successful cases of population-based behaviour change in the history of public health. This is made clear by a comparison with the decades of far less effective interventions under the 'old public health' model in attempts to control sexually transmitted diseases, cigarette smoking, poor nutrition, etc. The community-based dissemination of safer sex and safe use messages, which had been socially and culturally adapted to specific target groups, has proved the feasibility, effectiveness and efficiency of the 'new public health' and its superiority over former methods of control and containment. The behavioural changes, which are extensive and sustainable in both the mainly affected groups and in the public at large, can probably be improved even more if methods are further developed (Bochow *et al.*, 1994; Dubois-Arber *et al.*, 1997a, 1997b; Lagrange *et al.*, 1997). Primary prevention of HIV infection is based today on a broad foundation of knowledge in the fields of sexual science, behavioural science, milieu sociology, evaluation research, etc., illustrating what a large contribution social science research can make to rendering prevention policies more effective (Rosenbrock, 1995b).

Generalisation of this success to the prevention of other health risks is hindered not only by a lack of political will, but also and above all by the fact it is difficult to clarify the factors which led to success. What was the respective importance of each of the following?:

- the combined use of general and target group-specific campaigns
- the quality of the messages and their means of communication
- the social climate of acceptance for people with HIV/AIDS
- the social cohesion in the groups affected
- the influence of personal contact with people with HIV/AIDS.

Empirical research is confronted with the fact that practically all the 'tools' have been employed simultaneously. That is why it is possible to measure only their overall effect, with a number of methodological restrictions (Dubois-Arber *et al.*, 1997a, 1997b; Carael *et al.*, 1997; Pott, Chapter 6).

In addition, conceptual and practical problems for normalisation exist when it comes to expanding these successes to other areas of prevention. These problems can be found at five levels.

Level 1   If the risk of contracting a disease is distributed unevenly in a population, there is always the question whether prevention should be directed at the public at large or selectively at the groups primarily affected. In the first case it may be possible to avoid discrimination and to facilitate learning in general, but the primarily affected groups may receive inadequate information, and fear in the general population may be raised unnecessarily. On the other hand, the argument for concentrating efforts on the public at large is the fact that, because of their large numbers, the risk in the general population can over time exceed the risk among the primarily affected groups (Rose, 1992).

This prevention policy dilemma was aggravated in the case of HIV by the fact that the risk to gays, IV drug users and sex workers greatly exceeded that of the general population. They were also groups with a long history of discrimination. In the course of normalisation in Germany the pragmatic consequence was education for the general public being conducted by the government (through the Federal Centre for Health Education) and prevention for the primarily affected groups being delegated to state-financed AIDS service organisations. The experience with HIV makes clear that prevention policy decisions cannot be made on the basis of abstract epidemiological risk calculations alone, but require pragmatic adaptation to the national culture. In the case of HIV prevention this has meant, above all, adapting to perceptions of sex, drugs, and minorities.

Level 2   From the very beginning of the epidemic it has been easier to formulate appropriate prevention policy than to implement it. A substantial hindrance is the moralisation of the AIDS risk. However, the normalisation of AIDS in Germany has led to greater latitude for public communication about homosexuality, promiscuity and extramarital sex (Wellings and Field, 1996).

Level 3   In accordance with the philosophy of the WHO Ottawa Charter (1986) and for practical reasons, community-based prevention is dependent on ongoing voluntary commitment from the respective communities. Public authorities in Germany have sought to promote volunteering by providing state support. These resources have made possible the stabilisation and professionalisation of the AIDS service organisations. This has, however, led to ongoing tension between the desire for autonomy and a factual dependence, between voluntary and paid work, and between the levels of planning and implementation. The number of self-help organisations for gays, IV drug users, and sex workers rose very dramatically in Germany in the exceptionalist phase and has largely remained stable in the course of normalisation. However, there has been competition at the organisational level between the various tasks, with primary prevention being pitted against psychosocial and legal services in terms of time and resources.

Several hitherto inadequately answered questions are posed during the process of normalisation for community-based and target group specific prevention:

- What lobby, within the scope of a 'welfare mix' (Evers and Olk, 1996), is needed to sustain politically the volunteer-based services in times of tighter budgets and declining exceptionalism?
- What mix of incentives is required to recruit, train and retain an adequate corps of motivated volunteers?
- How can we counteract the tendency of self-help organisations to concentrate on the relatively easy-to-reach members of target groups while neglecting hard-to-reach populations?

Level 4   It is precisely the last question that is becoming increasingly thorny. At first, homosexual men from the more mobile and autonomous middle and upper classes appeared to be most impacted by HIV and AIDS. The first generation of prevention activists, drawn mainly from this group, not only tackled prevention for its own community but also helped implement prevention for the less well-organised IV drug users. Despite numerous important efforts to reverse the trend, AIDS prevention has increasingly become an event by middle-class gays for middle-class gays, with an additional bias in favour of men patronising the commercial subculture. This systematic deficit in community activities was tackled only hesitantly by the social scientists occupied with questions of prevention; therefore, it is not surprising that the variety and differentiation of prevention approaches has not addressed differences based on socio-economic status within the target groups (Luger, 1998).

This deficit is starting to take its revenge, since new HIV infections are increasingly occurring with disproportionate frequency in the lower classes in Germany (Bochow, Chapter 12; Marcus, Chapter 3). This stratification of sickness by social class poses the same policy questions for HIV as it does for other diseases. These questions related to social inequality and health outcomes are just beginning to be addressed in practical and scientific terms (Luger, 1998).

Level 5   Competing with these efforts is a re-medicalisation of HIV policy leading to a neglect of primary prevention and a renewed interest in early detection and treatment (secondary prevention), or even post exposure prophylaxis. This implies intervention targeted to the individual (that is, the HIV antibody test). The return to screening, case finding and compulsory partner notification and treatment is frequently called a return to proven principles of public health (for example, Burr, 1997; Gostin *et al.*, 1997; Lazzarani, 1998; more critical: Colfax and Bindman, 1998; opposed: Horton, 1998), as if the 'new public health' were not an improvement over the 'old public health' but the betrayal of unshakeable principles of public health as a whole. Without any adequate evidence (Gill, 1998; Gill *et al.*, 1998) HIV antibody tests are once again claimed to have a preventive, behavioural effect, a maximum number of HIV tests being viewed as a kind of indicator for effective prevention.   It is hardly ever recalled that a very large number of human lives could be saved if the resources required for tests would instead be invested in primary prevention (Gill, 1998).

The decision in favour of the basic model of AIDS prevention policy was made both for reasons of efficiency and for the protection of civil rights. This prevention model currently represents what is probably the most effective and efficient way to fight diseases that are mainly transmitted by sexual contact, an approach that will not become obsolete due to drugs being available to lengthen people's lives, minorities not having yet been subjected to witch hunts, and affected communities having been integrated into the political process. So far this debate has not assumed forms in any European country, including Germany, that could do any harm to testing policy, and by extension, to prevention policy.

To summarise the deficits outlined here: the participatory, community and communication oriented prevention model of publicly organised learning must be viewed as an endangered innovation. This danger becomes more acute in a phase in which primary prevention requires further development in conceptual terms. In view of the new therapeutic hopes, assessments of the magnitude of risks associated with an HIV infection might decline and thus a motive for preventive behaviour be weakened (Adam *et al.*, 1998; Hubert *et al.* 1998a, 1998b).

The risk of a failure would have a double impact: on HIV prevention and on the modernisation of prevention policy in general in industrialised countries, including Germany. In the debates centred on the HIV antibody test, for one, standards have been set in respect to its effectiveness and efficiency with regard to the desirable and undesirable effects of early detection (secondary prevention), standards that are still waiting to be applied to screenings for other diseases (Holland and Stewart, 1990; Miller and Lipman, 1996). For another, the most promising strategy of preventing diseases is at stake, namely, the model of publicly organised learning.

AIDS and drugs: the exception becomes the norm

Long before AIDS, the politics regarding narcotics in Germany, including IV drug use in particular, comprised a relatively independent arena in which the respective professional networks, institutions and regulatory bodies from the fields of health, social welfare, youth and criminal justice overlapped. Since the 1970s there have been two primary contradictory policy approaches in competition with each other: Repression and abstinence versus harm reduction. It is evident that the model of prevention adopted regarding the sexual transmission of HIV is only compatible with the harm reduction approach to drug use. In Germany, an already liberal drug policy was therefore expanded and stabilised under the influence of the AIDS crisis, bringing about a change in policy. (See Barsch, Chapter 14.)

A closer look at the transformation of drug policies in the context of AIDS yields the following picture. In the phase of policy formulation and emerging exceptionalism the drug policy existing prior to AIDS was essentially continued.

In the phase in which exceptionalism was consolidated, more liberal programs were formulated and, for the most part, also implemented. In the phase distinguished by a dwindling exceptionalism an ever broader liberal consensus gradually gained acceptance in drug policy. The normalisation triggered by AIDS had taken on a life of its own with the harm reduction coalitions gaining decisive strength because of AIDS.

While drug users in Germany can hope for more realistic, humane and effective treatment as a result of the AIDS crisis, the new possibilities of medical treatment for HIV are leading to new problems for this group. Whereas, the liberal drug policy can claim its first successes in the reduction of HIV risk (Pant, 1998; Uchtenhagen, 1995), the new combination therapies require an unusually high degree of adherence to treatment which is difficult to reconcile with the real life situation of many drug users, homeless people and sex workers. New outreach strategies are called for which integrate medical and social care; current health care structures typically require people needing help to arrange an office visit. The 'normal' medical care of drug-using patients therefore does not reflect the positive developments having taken place in drug policies themselves. Rather, there is the threat that the 'normally poor course of health policy' (Rosenbrock, 1986) will continue for this population, thus leading to further discrimination of an already marginalised group of patients.

Conclusion

In Germany the rise of AIDS led to important and profound innovations in the fields of prevention, patient care, health policy and civil rights. Compared with the usually sluggish and incremental reactions to other health-related problems, these innovations can be called exceptional. This exception from the normally poor course of events taken by health policies can be explained for the most part by the political thrust resulting from a general fear in society of an impending health catastrophe and a loss of civil rights. As a consequence, an alliance of health professionals, social movements and persons affected by the disease made political use of the latitude resulting from a lack of effective therapies.

The predicted disaster failed to materialise. The reasons for this are to be found not only in initial overestimates of the risks, but also in the prevention policy and civil rights successes of the exceptionalist alliance. The degree to which exceptionalism is being institutionalised and codified in law will largely determine the direction and extent of further normalisation. Currently, it is not so much the lack of ideas as much as a lack of strength hindering a second wave of innovations which could consolidate the exceptionalist model in prevention and patient care, more generally (Schaeffer, 1995b).

In this respect three basic forms of normalisation are emerging in this as yet incomplete process.

In part, policies developed within the scope of exceptionalism are being generalised (normalisation as generalisation). In the field of patient care, for example, the application of the principle 'outpatient before inpatient', the development of community-based and disease-specific services, as well as patient-friendly structures led to innovations that had a 'contagious' effect on the care of other groups of patients.

In other areas the special handling of AIDS is being institutionalised (normalisation as stabilisation). This can be seen, for instance, in the disease-specific services still left in patient care, the institutionalisation of target group-specific HIV primary prevention, and also in changes in the definition of tasks and structures of public health institutions.

Certain programs and institutions that gave rise to exceptionalism are being cut back to the prior status quo (normalisation as regression). For example, numerous specialised organisational units in government and public health institutions are being dissolved or reintegrated into general structures. What is particularly dangerous in terms of health policy in Germany is the reduction in absolute terms of funds going to the primary prevention of HIV.

Finally, in view of the global AIDS crisis, it is evident that Germany has failed as much as most other wealthy countries. It is neither humane nor a sign of action in the direction of globalisation and sustainability when in 1997 only some 10 per cent of the world resources were available to developing countries in which about 90 per cent of HIV infections occur (Morin, 1998). Despite many official declarations and numerous attempts to the contrary, there has never been any exceptional status accorded to AIDS in regard to the international distribution of resources, making AIDS like any of the myriad diseases which ravage the developing world without adequate intervention.

Notes

1   For reasons of clarity, the terminology and sequence of this description are oriented to the phases/stages of the public health action cycle (National Academy of Sciences, 1988; Rosenbrock, 1995a). The general criticism of the action cycle also holds true for AIDS: this model inherently constricts the political process to the perception and actions of one single, powerful actor (implicitly the respective central government, in most cases) (Héritier, 1993). The model thus cannot reproduce the complexity of issue communities generating governance structures with a great many governmental and non-governmental actors. The analytical benefit of the model is, therefore, to be found mainly in its use as 'phase heuristics' (Sabatier and Jenkins-Smith, 1993).

2   In Germany, federal support for social science research did not begin until five years after the funding for biomedical research. At no point in time did the social science expenditures account for more than a tenth of the total public spending on AIDS research (Kießling and Vettermann, 1995). Research funding is lacking for health policy, as well, including for research on applying innovations in AIDS work to other areas of health care, thereby limiting the dissemination of knowledge. Patient care research has been particularly neglected. A professionally managed transfer of knowledge, which would be a necessary precondition for the dissemination and continuation of innovation (Rogers, 1983), can hardly be expected in such a situation.

3   Maximisation of the number of people tested for HIV antibodies, accompanied by the hope of effective primary prevention, was also the main argument for approval of home test kits in the US (Philips *et al.*, 1995). These hopes were not fulfilled, of course, the sales figures remaining far below expectations (Karcher, 1997; Robert Koch Institut, 1997). In Europe this technical innovation is viewed with a critical eye, mainly because

there is no evidence for improving the efficiency of primary prevention and because the possibility of pre- and post-test counseling is lost as a result (Rosenbrock, 1997) Therefore, the HIV home test has not yet been approved in Europe.

References

Abholz, H. H. (1994) 'Grenzen medizinischer Prävention', in R. Rosenbrock, H. Kühn and B. Köhler (eds), *Präventionspolitik. Gesellschaftliche Strategien der Gesundheitssicherung*, Berlin: edition sigma: 54–82.

Adam, P. *et al.* (1998) 'HIV/AIDS preventive attitudes and behaviour of French and Swiss gay men in the era of new treatments: a comparison of two national surveys', Poster 34107 presented at the oral communication no. 642, 12th World AIDS Conference, Geneva.

Aust, B. (1996) *Berufliche Gratifikationskrisen im Dienstleistungsbereich.* Unpublished report of Project D2. Dusseldorf.

Ballard, J. (1998) 'The constitution of aids in Australia: taking 'government at a distance' seriously', in B. Hindess and M. Dean (eds), *Governing Australia*, Melbourne: Cambridge University Press: 125–38.

Bayer, R. (1989) *Private Acts, Social Consequences, AIDS and the Politics of Public Health*, New York and London: Free Press/Collier Macmillan.

—— (1991) 'Public health policy and the AIDS epidemic: an end to HIV exceptionalism?' *JAMA* 324: 1500–4.

Bayer, R. and Oppenheimer, G. M. (1998) 'AIDS death and impotence: Doctors confront the limits of medicine', in *Working Papers for Synthesis Sessions of the 2nd European Conference 'AIDS in Europe. New Challenges for Social and Behavioural Sciences'*, UNESCO, 12–15 January, Paris.

Bochow, M., Chiarotti, F., Davies, P., Dubois-Arber, F., Dür, W., Fouchard, J., Gruet, F., McManus, T., Markert, S., Sandfort, T. *et al.* (1994) 'Sexual behaviour of gay and bisexual men in eight European countries', *AIDS Care* 6(5): 533–459.

Boom, F. van den (1998) 'The normalisation of AIDS? AIDS policies: comparison, changes and perspectives', in *Working Papers for Synthesis Sessions of the 2nd European Conference 'AIDS in Europe. New Challenges for Social and Behavioural Sciences'*, UNESCO, 12–15 January, Paris.

Brandt, A. M. (1987) *No Magic Bullet: A Social History of Venereal Disease in the United States*, New York: Oxford University Press.

Burr, C. (1997) 'The AIDS exception: privacy *vs.* public health', *Atlantic Monthly* 279(6): 67.

Carael, M., Buvé, A. and Awusabo-Asare, K. (1997) 'The making of HIV epidemics: what are the driving forces?' *AIDS* 11 (suppl B): S23–S31.

Cattacin, S. (1996) 'Organisatorische Probleme der HIV/AIDS-Politik in föderalen Staaten: Deutschland, Österreich und Schweiz im Vergleich', *Journal für Sozialforschung* 36(1): 73–85.

—— (1998) 'The organisational normalisation of unexpected events. the case of HIV/AIDS in perspective', in *Working Papers for Synthesis Sessions of the 2nd European Conference 'AIDS in Europe. New Challenges for Social and Behavioural Sciences'*, UNESCO, 12–15 January, Paris.

Colfax, G. N. and Bindman, A. B. (1998) 'Health benefits and risks of reporting HIV-infected individuals by name', *American Journal of Public Health* 88: 876–9.

Downs, A. (1972) 'Up and down with ecology – the "issue-attention cycle"', *Public Interest* 28: 38–50.

Dubois-Arber, F., Jeannin, A., Meystre-Agustoni, G., Moreau-Gruet, F., Haour-Knipe, M., Spencer, B. and Paccaud, F. (1997a) *Evaluation of the AIDS Prevention Strategy in Switzerland Mandated by the Federal Office of Public Health. Fifth Assessment Report 1993–1995,* Institut universitaire de médecine sociale et préventive, Cah. Rech. Doc. IUMSP, no. 120b.

Dubois-Arber, F., Jeannin, A., Konings, E. and Paccaud, F. (1997b) 'Increased condom use without major changes in sexual behaviour among the general population in Switzerland', *American Journal of Public Health* 87(4): 558–66.

Evers, A. and Olk, T. (1996) 'Wohlfahrtspluralismus – Analytische und normativ-politische Dimensionen eines Leitbegriffs,' in A. Evers and T. Olk (eds), *Wohlfahrtsplural-ismus: vom Wohlfahrtsstaat zur Wohlfahrtsgesellschaft,* Opladen: Westdeutscher Verlag: 9–62.

Farquhar, J. W., Fortmann, S., Flora, J. A. *et al.* (1990) 'Effects of Community Wide Education on Cardiovascular Disease Risk Factors: The Stanford Five-City Project', *JAMA* 264: 359–65.

Fee E. and Fox, D. M. (eds) (1992) *AIDS: The making of a chronic disease,* Berkeley, Calif.: University of California Press.

Frankenberg, G. (1992) 'Germany: the uneasy triumph of pragmatism', in D. Kirp and R. Bayer (eds), *AIDS in Industrial Democracies: Passions, Politics and Policies,* New Brunswick, N.J.: Rutgers University Press.

Gill, O. N. (1998) 'Promoting testing is no substitute for recognising risk', *British Medical Journal* 316: 295–6.

Gill, O. N., McGarrigle, C. A., MacDonald, N. D. and Sinka, K. (1998) 'UK HIV testing policy: results, changes and challenges – will 'normalisation' of HIV testing weaken, rather than strengthen, primary prevention?', *Working Papers for Synthesis Sessions of the 2nd European Conference 'Aids in Europe. New Challenges for Social and Behavioural Sciences',* UNESCO, 12–15 January, Paris.

Gostin, L., Ward, J. W. and Baker, C. A. (1997) 'National HIV case reporting for the United States', *New England Journal of Medicine* 337: 1162–7.

Hamouda, O., Nießing, W. and Voß, L. (1997) 'AIDS/HIV 1996. Bericht zur epidemi-ologi-schen Situation in der Bundesrepublik zum 31.12.1996,' *RKI-Hefte* (17), ed. RKI-AIDS-Zentrum, Berlin.

Héritier, A. (1993) 'Policy-Analyse. Elemente der Kritik und der Neuorientierung', in A. Héritier (ed.), *Policy Analyse. Kritik und Neuorientierung,* Opladen: Westdeutscher Verlag: 9–36.

Holland, W. W. and Stewart, S. (1990) *Screening in Health Care: Benefit or Blame?* London: Nuffield Provincial Hospital Trust.

Horton, M. (1998) 'Réactions, récidive et relations sans protection: la criminalisation croissante de la contamination par le VIH. ANRS. Le sida en Europe: nouveaux enjeux pour les sciences sociales', Collection Sciences Sociales et SIDA, Paris: *ANRS:* 35–42.

Hubert, M. *et al.* (1998a) 'Public awareness of the new treatments and changes in HIV risk perception: comparison of four European countries in 1997–98', Poster no 43573, Oral communication LB 16 at the 12th World AIDS Conference, Geneva.

Hubert, M., Bajos, N. and Sandfort, T. (eds). (1998b) *Sexual Behaviour and HIV/AIDS in Europe,* London: UCL Press.

Karcher, H. L. (1997) 'HIV home test kit banned in Germany', *British Medical Journal* 315: 627.

Kießling, S. and Vettermann, W. (1995) 'Effektivität staatlich geförderter Forschung – eine Analyse für den Bereich AIDS', *AIDS-Forschung* 10(5): 245–50.

Kingdon, J. (1984) *Agendas, Alternatives, and Public Policies,* Boston: Little, Brown.

Kirp, D. and Bayer, R. (eds) (1992) *AIDS in Industrial Democracies: Passions, Politics, and Policies*, New Brunswick, N.J.: Rutgers University Press.

Kleiber, D., Enzmann, D. and Gusy, B. (1995) 'Stress and burnout of health care professionals working with AIDS-patients', *International Journal of Health Sciences* 6: 96–101.

Lagrange, H., Lhomond, B., Calvez, M., Levinson, S., Maillochon, F., Mogoutov, A. and Warszawski, J. (1997) *L'entrée dans la sexualité. Le comportement des jeunes dans le contexte du sida*, Paris: Edition La Découverte.

Lazzarani, Z. (1998) 'Moving to national HIV reporting', Paper presented at the 12th World AIDS Conference, Oral Session C23, 30 June, Geneva.

Lichtenstein, B. (1997) 'Tradition and experiment in New Zealand AIDS policy', *AIDS and Public Policy Journal* 12(2): 79–87.

Luger, L. (1998) *HIV/AIDS Prevention and 'Class' and Socio-Economic Related Factors of Risk of HIV Infection*. Publications Series of the Research Unit Public Health Policy, P98–204, Berlin: Social Science Research Centre.

Mann, M. (1986) *The Sources of Social Power: vol. I – A History of Power from the Beginning to A.D. 1760*, Cambridge: Cambridge University Press.

Miller, R. and Lipman, M. (1996) 'HIV pre-test discussion. Not just for specialists', *British Medical Journal* 313(20): 130.

Moers, M. and Schaeffer, D. (1992a) 'Die Bedeutung niedergelassener Ärzte für die Herstellung von Versorgungskontinuität bei Patienten mit HIV-Symptomen', in D. Schaeffer, M. Moers and R. Rosenbrock (eds), *AIDS-Krankenversorgung*, Berlin: edition sigma: 133–60.

—— (1992b) 'Perspectives on a continuum of care for patients with HIV-symptons', in *Health systems – The challenge of change*. Proceedings of the 5th International Conference on System Science in Health Care, Prague: Omnipress: 1546–1549.

—— (1998) 'The impact of AIDS on nurses and nursing care', in *Working Papers for Synthesis Sessions of the 2nd European Conference 'AIDS in Europe. New Challenges for Social and Behavioural Sciences'*, UNESCO, 12–15 January, Paris.

Morin, S. (1998) 'North American Funding for HIV in the Developing World', Paper presented at the 12th World AIDS Conference, Geneva.

National Academy of Sciences; Institute of Medicine (1988) *The Future of Public Health*, Washington D.C.: National Academy of Sciences.

Pant, H. A. (1998) *HIV-Infektionen bei iv Drogenkonsumenten – Sozialepidemiologische Befunde zur Ätiologie durch Metaanalysen und Primärdatenanalysen*, Berlin: Freie Universität Berlin, Institut für Prävention und psychosoziale Gesundheitsforschung.

Philips, K. A., Flatt, S. F., Morrison, K. R. and Coates, T. J. (1995) 'Potential use of home HIV testing', *New England Journal of Medicine* 332: 1308–10.

Puska, P., Nissinen, A. and Tuomilehto, J. (1985) 'The community-based strategy to prevent coronary heart disease: conclusions from ten years of the North Karelia Project', *Annual Review of Public Health* 6: 147–93.

Robert Koch Institut (1997) 'InfFo-Diskussionsforum zur Frage HIV-Heim- bzw. HIV-Home-Collection-Test', *InfFo* 2: 35-44.

Rogers, E. M. (1983) *Diffusion of Innovation*, New York and London: Free Press.

Rose, G. (1992) *The Strategy of Preventive Medicine*, London: Oxford University Press.

Rosenbrock, R. (1986) *AIDS kann schneller besiegt werden – Gesundheitspolitik am Beispiel einer Infektionskrankheit* (3rd edn 1987), Hamburg: VSA Verlag.

—— (1987) 'Some social and health policy requirements for the prevention of AIDS', *Health Promotion* 2: 61–168.

—— (1991) 'Screening for human immunodeficiency virus', *International Journal of Technology Assessment in Health Care* 7(3): 263–74.

—— (1993) 'AIDS: Questions and lessons for public health', *AIDS and Public Policy Journal* 8(1): 5–19.

—— (1994a) 'Die Normalisierung von AIDS, teils nach vorne, teils zurück', in D. Kirp and R. Bayer (eds), *Strategien gegen AIDS. Ein internationaler Politikvergleich*, Berlin: edition sigma: 480–501.

—— (1994b) 'Der HIV-Test ist die Antwort – aber auf welche Fragen? Vom Nutzen einer Diagnose für Prävention und Therapie', in R. Rosenbrock, H. Kühn and B. Köhler (eds), *Präventionspolitik. Gesellschaftliche Strategien der Gesundheitssicherung*, Berlin: edition sigma: 358–82.

—— (1995a) 'Public Health als soziale Innovation', *Das Gesundheitswesen* 57(3): 140–4.

—— (1995b) 'Social sciences and HIV/AIDS policies: experiences and perspectives', in D. Friedrich and W. Heckmann (eds), *AIDS in Europe – The Behavioural Aspect*, vol. 1, Berlin: edition sigma: 259–69.

—— (1997) 'Welche Verbesserungen kann der HIV-Home Sampling Test bringen?', *Infektionsepidemiologische Forschung* 2: 40–3.

Rosewitz, B. and Webber, D. (1990) *Reformversuche und Reformblockaden im deutschen Gesundheitswesen*, Frankfurt/Main and New York: Campus Verlag.

Rucht, D. (1994) Modernisierung und neue soziale Bewegungen, Frankfurt/Main and New York: Campus.

Sabatier, P. and Jenkins-Smith, H. (1993) *Policy Change and Learning: An Advocacy Coalition Approach*, Boulder, Colo.: Westview Press.

Schaeffer, D. (1995a) 'Patientenorientierte Krankenversorung: AIDS als Herausforderung', *Zeitschrift für Gesundheitswissenschaften* 3(4): 332–48.

Schaeffer, D. (1995b) 'AIDS and innovations in the German health care system', *International Journal of Health Science* 6(2): 77–84.

Schaeffer D. (1996) 'Innovationsprozesse in der ambulanten Pflege. AIDS als Pilotprojekt,' *Pflege: Die wissenschaftliche Zeitung für Pflegeberufe* 9(2): 140–9.

Schaeffer, D., Moers, M. and Rosenbrock, R. (eds) (1992) *AIDS-Krankenversorgung. Ergebnisse sozialwissenschaftlicher AIDS-Forschung* vol. 8, Berlin: edition sigma.

Setbon, M. (1993) *Pouvoirs contre sida. De la transfusion sanguine au dépistage: Décisions et pratiques en France, Grande-Bretagne et Suède*, Paris: Seuil.

Uchtenhagen, A. (1995) 'Harm reduction: The case of Switzerland', *European Addict Research* 1: 86–91.

Ullrich, A. (1987) *Krebsstation. Belastungen der Helfer. Eine empirische Studie in Bayern*, Frankfurt/Main.

Wellings, K. and Field, B. (1996) *Stopping AIDS. AIDS/HIV Public Education and the Mass Media in Europe*, London, and New York: Longman.

WHO (1986) *Ottawa Charter for Health Promotion*, Geneva: World Health Organisation.

Index

Milton Keynes UK
Ingram Content Group UK Ltd.
UKHW031146141024
449569UK00024B/1022